DENTAL OFFICE ADMINISTRATION IN THE CANADIAN HEALTHCARE SYSTEM

PROF. USHA DABAS
Director, Healthcare Faculty

SPRINGFIELD COLLEGE OF HEALTHCARE, MGMT & TECH

ISBN: 9798494079459

CONTENTS

PREFACE

With the current developments and introduction of the most advanced dental materials, techniques and technologies, the field of dentistry has undergone radical and tremendous changes during the past couple of decades. Globally, more and more people have already started generating interest and inclination towards the practice of dental surgery, opting for the practice of dentistry as a professional career. This is certainly due to the increasing responsiveness and demand for the sophisticated services with the increasing dental awareness and knowledge of oral and dental diseases. Of course, the significant role has been played by other factors such as paying capacity of the people and improving economy of the various developing countries, due to which more and more people believe in quality dental treatment. Moreover, the young people of newer generation consider the concept of care, cosmetic and conservation which in true sense is the very domain of the field of modern-day dentistry practice.

As a matter of fact, to serve the community better and advance the realm of Oral and Dental Science, many institutions too have joined in this global endeavor of spreading the knowledge and expertise of the subject of Dental surgery by constituting various courses in the different specialties of dentistry.

This book is regarded by the author as an introduction to modern dentistry and its fundamental concepts obligatory to an accurate dental practice. The text is written primarily to aid dental staff members, who are not merely engaged but truly serve as the essential segment of the modern-day dental practice such as dental administrators, dental hygienists, dental technicians, dental nurses and dental surgery assistants. This book deals from the fundamental and historical background of the dentistry to the current trends and future of the dentistry. All the concepts are compiled to highlight the most recent advancements in the sphere of Oral and dental science. This book will be very useful for all those who have ever desired and cherished to learn the fundamentals and perceptions of dentistry as well as participate as an effective team member in the dental office. It will also provide guidance to the new entrants to understand the subject of Oral and dental science thoroughly, faster and more effectively.

CHAPTER 1
DENTAL HISTORY

EARLY TIMES

Oral disease has been a problem for humans from the beginning of history. Skulls of Cro-Magnon peoples, who inhabited the earth 25,000 years ago, show evidence of tooth decay. The earliest recorded reference to oral disease is from an ancient (5000 BC) Sumerian text that describes, "tooth worms" as a cause of dental decay. There is historical evidence that the Chinese used acupuncture around 2700 BC to treat pain associated with tooth decay.

The history of dentistry dates back thousands of years to ancient civilizations. Evidence of this history is available through archeological excavations. Archeologists have been able to date dentistry as far back as 3000 B.C. One example of early dental care is found in human skulls which include various forms of tooth replacement as well as other dental procedures. In addition to actual remains, 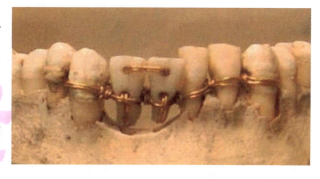 scientists have discovered dental tools such as forceps and dental picks. It is interesting when we realize that many of the designs of these ancient artifacts are utilized in the instruments today. In many civilizations such as those of the Chinese, the Egyptians, and the Greeks, there were designated healers who experimented in the treatment of dental ailments. Let us take a closer look at these ancient healers and the accomplishments they made in the world of dentistry.

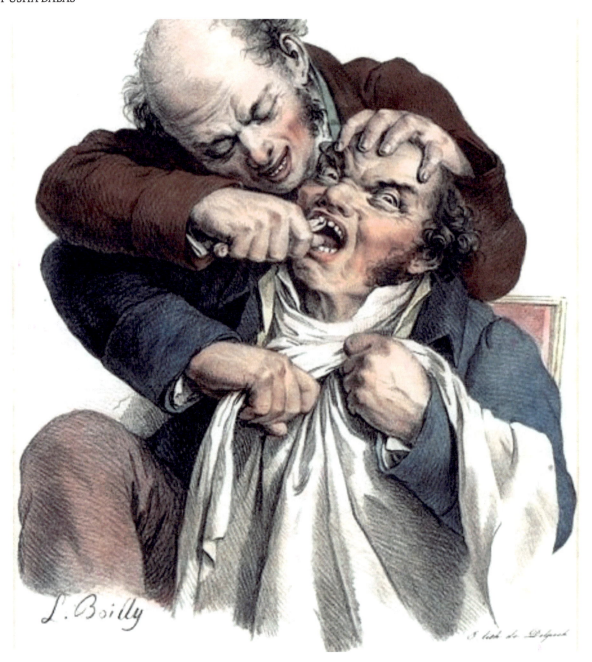

L. Boilly

The Egyptians

One of the greatest civilizations of ancient times was the Egyptians. There was a well-defined class system in Egypt. Those within the upper hierarchy often proved to become extraordinary in their field. The system helped to produce some of the most accomplished architects, scientists, and healers. The ancient Egyptians excelled in many areas of science, one of these being dentistry. Historians have been able to determine that one of the earliest dentists in ancient Egypt was Hesi-Re, who lived about 3,100–2,181 B.C. during the reign of Zoser. It is felt that he was one of the greatest scientists of his time to be solely concerned with the treatment of dental pain. It is believed that the Egyptians experienced all of the major dental diseases, including *caries* (cavities) and *periodontal* (gum) disease. However, they also suffered from rather unique types of dental problems due to their culture. The basic diet of the Egyptians consisted mainly of herbivorous plants and breads. The bread was made of grains, which were ground on rough stones. This method caused small stones to become incorporated into the bread dough. Unfortunately, they had no means of extracting these stones and they were baked into the bread. This produced a bread which was very coarse in consistency and difficult to chew, without causing dental problems. The rest of their diet consisted mainly of plants. However, as the area in which the Egyptians lived was very sandy, the plants were quite gritty. This situation caused yet another dental problem. The combination of these two conditions caused extensive wear and *attrition* (weakening) of their teeth. This led to problems such as nerve exposure and abscesses. The main dental work available to the ancient Egyptians consisted of extractions and management of dental abscesses. They did not put a high priority on either oral hygiene or preventive care. Archeologists have never located any type of a toothbrush or dental cleaning device at an Egyptian site. Their main concern appears to have been the treatment of ailments after the onset of disease. It's also interesting to discover that the Egyptians seemed to place more emphasis on some of their dental care after death. Historians have learned that the replacement of teeth by artificial means seemed to be accomplished only after death. The Egyptians used to mummify their corpses. However, before this was done, the body was to be as intact as possible, including the replacement of missing teeth. They believed that this ritual helped to repair the person for the afterlife.

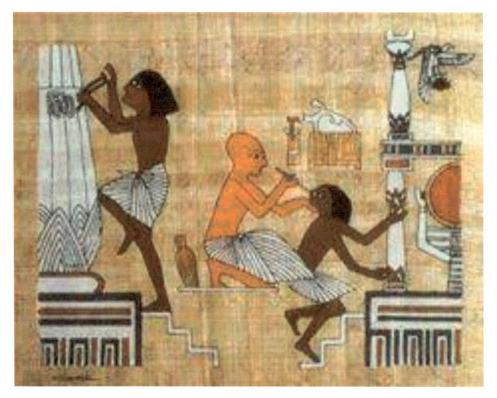

Among the papyri of ancient Egypt is the Ebers papyrus, which throws light on medical practices. It was written between 1700 and 1500 BC and contains material dating back as far as 3700 BC. The Papyrus Ebers contains references to diseases of the teeth, as well as prescriptions for substances such as olive oil, dates, onions, beans, and green lead, to be mixed and applied "against the throbbing of the bennut blisters in the teeth." An Egyptian lower jaw, dated by experts from 2900 to 2750 BC, demonstrates two holes drilled through the bone, presumably to drain an abscessed tooth. Much of early dentistry was practiced

The Phoenicians

The Phoenicians were an ancient civilization that occupied the area known today as Syria and Lebanon. Theirs was a culture that consisted mainly of traders. These ancient seamen traveled the Mediterranean Basin and through these explorations gained much insight and knowledge into various technologies. The beginnings of several dental technologies can be found in the Phoenician civilization. Their contemporaries, the Egyptians, influenced much of their knowledge of dentistry. One such example is in a treatment of periodontal disease. The Egyptians utilized a technique for treating teeth affected by periodontal disease where the mobile teeth were splinted (fixed together). The Phoenicians took this technique and refined it. Skulls have been found in archeological digs, which demonstrate periodontally compromised teeth that have been splinted with gold arch wire. This technique utilized by the Phoenicians isn't, unlike the techniques preferred by some dentists today. The Phoenicians also experimented in bridgework. Several examples of fixed bridgework have been found in skulls unearthed during archeological digs. The method used consists of ivory-carved false teeth attached to natural teeth by thin gold wire. This is yet another example of the knowledge of the Phoenicians and its effect on the beginnings of dentistry. Other ancient civilizations were fortunate, as the knowledge of the Phoenicians was passed on, thus making them a major vessel in the advancement of dental awareness and technology.

The Greeks

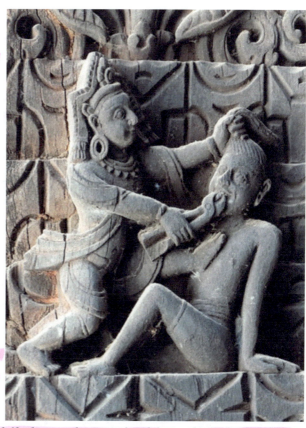

The ancient Greeks lived and flourished in an age of discovery. It was during the time of this civilization that there was much advancement made in the field of medicine. The earliest of these advancements was found in the fifth century B.C. A medical school located on the Isle of Cos and Cnidus was the centerpiece of discovery at that time. The Greeks were firm believers in the worship of various gods. Much of the medicine that was practiced at this time was based on the worship of Asclepius, the Greek god of healing and medicine. The way a toothache was treated was also based on this belief. A patient with a toothache was brought to a priest for medical treatment. The first phase of the treatment was a form of relaxation. The patient was given a sleep-inducing potion that helped to bring him or her into a state of relaxation. The priest would visit the patient while he or she was in this semi wakeful sleep. He would instruct the patient on a course of treatment. If the treatment were successful, the patient would have to make some type of tribute to the healing temple. The tribute generally took the form of stone tablets carved in the shape of the afflicted body part, in this case a tooth. The tablets would have writing carved into them with words praising Asclepius. It's interesting to note that numerous stones carved in the shape of teeth have been found at archeological digs at ancient temples.

The Greek civilization is also noted for its development of an alternative method of medicine known as the Hippocratic method. This method was named after a man who was known as the father of modern medicine, Hippocrates. The method, which Hippocrates utilized in treating patients, was one of observation. He would observe the ailments of his patients and then treat them rationally and systematically. He based all states of disease and health on the balance of what he termed *cardinal humors* and *elemental conditions.*

Hippocrates believed that the cardinal humors consisted of four bodily fluids—blood, phlegm, black bile, and yellow bile. In conjunction with these were the four elemental conditions—cold, hot, dry, and moist. He believed that the perfect balance of these eight states meant physical wellness for the patient. An unbalance of any of these resulted in disease. Different unbalances were related to different diseases of the body. Hippocrates's observation of his patient in relation to these balances and unbalances was his method of treating patients. Hippocrates is also known for the research and books he wrote about the maladies of the teeth and mouth. He believed that all dental problems were related to a natural inherited weakness of the body. He was against the use of extractions as a treatment unless a tooth was loose and, therefore, unable to be saved. Carious (decayed) teeth, he thought, should be treated symptomatically and not removed. Hippocrates and Aristotle wrote of ointments and cautery with a red-hot wire to treat diseases of the teeth and oral tissues. They also spoke of tooth extraction and the use of wires to stabilize jaw fractures or bind loose teeth.

The medical field flourished throughout the ages as a result of Hippocrates's teachings. The learning of arts and sciences continued under the rule of Alexander the Great into the third century B.C. Evidence of this has been discovered in archeological sites in recent years. Another famous Greek physician named Claudius Galen is noteworthy. His lifespan was from A.D. 120 to A.D. 199. He is best known for his writings on medical advances during his era. Part of his medical writing included information on dentistry and dental anatomy. It is in Galen's writings that we find documentation that teeth are made of bone. It was his belief that, since teeth are exposed, they must contain nerves within their structure. This, then, would protect the teeth from damage due to mechanical use. It is interesting that this premise of Galen's is still maintained today.

The Chinese

Ancient China is responsible for contributing much to the modern world. Specifically, this civilization introduced many innovations to the field of dentistry. The Chinese developed several methods of treating tooth disease, many before western European countries utilized them. For example, they began treating toothaches with arsenic about A.D. 1000. They are also noted for their development of using silver amalgam for filling teeth. Another area in which the Chinese were very astute is the field of oral medicine. The Chinese were particularly advanced in their observation of the oral cavity. In an ancient work called the *Canon of Medicine,* dentistry is discussed. A section of this work is dedicated specifically to *mastication* (chewing) and *deglutition* (swallowing). The Chinese were also interested in systemic diseases and their connection to oral manifestations. For example, they recognized that prior to the development of measles, white spots would appear in a person's oral cavity. Another significant area of study among Chinese surgeons was oral surgery. Scientists have discovered many writings regarding the extraction of teeth and the instruments utilized to perform such tasks. In addition, information has been found relating to the abscesses of teeth and other oral structures. The Chinese based many treatments for abscesses on scientific observation. Finally, the Chinese surgeons delved extensively into surgery techniques of the oral cavity. For example, there's written documentation regarding tumor removal and surgical repair due to trauma. They also dealt extensively with early repair of cleft palates (opening in the roof of the mouth), lip, and other congenital defects.

The Romans

The ancient Roman civilization is an excellent source for information relating to the lifestyles of ancient times. We are fortunate to benefit from the writings of Roman scientists and scholars, as it is from these works that we are able to learn from this civilization. There was a scholar who lived about A.D. 30 named Celsus. He created a medical documentation called *On Medicine,* which is considered to be one of the best medical works of its time. It is interesting to note that although his work has served as one of the first medical texts, Celsus wasn't a physician. Celsus wrote in his book on several areas of dentistry. One subject of interest to him was in the induction of sleep for patients who suffered from toothaches. He also wrote quite a bit on the treatment to aid in the resolution of pain from dental abscesses. The writing of Celsus also contained documentation regarding the first recognized cases of orthodontic treatment. This was accomplished through the use of appliances and finger pressure.

The Arabians

Arabian physicians attached great importance to clean teeth. They described various procedures to "scrape" the teeth and designed sets of specialized instruments to accomplish that task. The Arabians using a "toothbrush," a small polishing stick that was beaten and softened at one end, applied mouthwashes and dentifrice powders.

THE MIDDLE AGES

The Middle Ages, for the most part, was a time of stagnation as far as dental history is concerned. Medical advancements seemed to come to a complete standstill. Dental advances during this time were almost absent, with a few noted exceptions. This dry spell continued until the days of the Renaissance. Though the advances were limited, there were some notable discoveries during the Middle Ages. One of the most

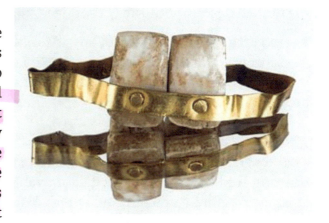

prominent was by a physician named Scrapion who lived during the tenth century. This physician, through his research, accurately described the number of roots found on particular teeth. He also correctly hypothesized the reasoning behind why teeth contain a different number of roots. It was his opinion that lower molars only required two roots due to their strong jaw support. He also noted that, in contrast, upper molars required three roots as they have less jaw support. Another noted dental figure during the Middle Ages was Abulcasis. He was a resident of Spain and lived between 1045 and 1120 A.D. He noted the necessity of oral hygiene. He wrote many works on the subject of cleaning teeth. These works included the importance of oral hygiene and the consequences of not following it. Abulcasis also wrote a list of his opinion of the rules to be followed for completing dental extractions. This did, however, include his opinion that any tooth extraction should only be done as a last resort.

Throughout the Middle Ages in Europe, physicians or surgeons who would go to the patient's homemade dentistry available to wealthier individuals. Decay would sometimes be removed from teeth with a "dental drill," a metal rod that was rotated between the palms. Soft filling materials provided short-term alleviation of discomfort by keeping air from the open cavity. Dentistry for poorer people took place in the marketplace, where self-taught vagabonds would extract teeth for a small fee.

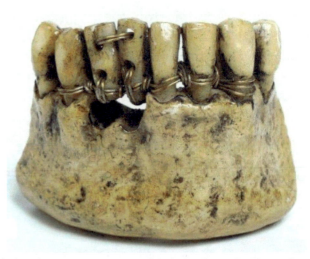

From the Middle Ages to the early 1700s much dental therapy was provided by so called "barber surgeons." These jacks-of-all-trades would not only extract teeth and perform minor surgery, but they also cut hair, applied leeches to let blood, and performed embalming.

Italian sources from the 1400s mention the use of gold leaf as dental filling material. Later, the French described the use of soft lead fillings to repair teeth after decay was removed.

There's little documentation of any advances in the dental field during the rest of the Middle Ages. It was not until the dawn of the Renaissance that any medical discoveries flourished. It was during this time that the study of dentistry became a separate science among the prestigious scientists of the day.

The Renaissance

The Renaissance was a time of rediscovery and technological advancement. Methods of printing information advanced as movable type became available, thus making it easier than ever before to record and spread knowledge. Scholars were now able to share their discoveries through the printed word. Many great scientists of medicine emerged during this period. One of the most noted was Andreas Vesalius (1510–1560). His works were so far advanced for his time that he is considered the father of modern anatomy. His main contribution to the field of dentistry is in mastication. He discovered that teeth all have a different pattern of bite called occlusion. A contemporary of Vesalius was Pasé, who is considered to be the father of modern surgery. He lived in France during the mid-1500s. He made several notable advancements in the field of gunshot wounds and reconstruction. He was one of the first surgeons to create artificial limbs. Pasé also had many accomplishments in the study of dentistry with specific regard to reconstruction. He produced artificial teeth to replace those lost due to trauma and periodontal disease. He is also known for his creation of a device utilized to close the opening left by a cleft palate. A cleft palate is congenital in nature and can extend into the patient's nasal sinus causing difficulties in eating and swallowing. The device Pasé invented is considered to be the first fabricated *obturator* (a device made to block the opening in the cleft palate). Pasé is also recognized for some of his writings. He wrote extensively on tooth extractions and methods of tooth reimplantation after a tooth has been *evulsed* (torn away) by acute trauma. Once dentistry became an established field, much significant advancement was made in the field. Pierre Fauchard (1678-1761), a French surgeon, is credited with being the "father of modem dentistry". His book, *The Surgeon Dentist- A Treatise on Teeth,* describes the basic oral anatomy and function, signs and symptoms of oral pathology, operative methods for removing decay and restoring teeth, periodontal disease (pyorrhea), orthodontics, replacement of missing teeth, and tooth transplantation.

Fauchard published many of his works during the early to mid-1700s. His writings are some of the most important publications in dentistry even today. It was his opinion that dentists should be recognized as specialists separate from medical doctors and should hold the title *surgeon dentists.* This title is still utilized in France today. Fauchard's writings were quite involved for his time. He included detailed descriptions of treatment advances. He also produced detailed drawings and descriptions of instruments used. Fauchard's interests included all facets of dentistry. In fact, he was the first to contradict Galen's theory of tooth worm (cavities caused by tooth worms). He believed that cavities were formed by physical actions rather than the presence of tooth worm. Other areas about which he wrote included the importance of dental hygiene. He also wrote about his experiments with filling cavities with tin or lead. He used the treatment of filling teeth for cosmetic reasons. Fauchard fabricated several types of tooth replacement devices. He made bridges using gold wire in ivory teeth for limited tooth replacement. He also created many designs of full dentures using gold, ivory teeth, and springs for retention. He also did some experimentation with the replacement of traumatically evulsed teeth (teeth torn out by a trauma, such as an accident). Fauchard`s text was followed by others that continued to expand the knowledge of the profession throughout Europe. Two popular books, Natural History of Human Teeth (1771) and Practical Treatise on the Diseases of the Teeth (1778), were written by English physiologist John Hunter, surgeon general to the British army. John Hunter took the beginnings of the practice of tooth replacement from Fauchard and built upon it. Hunter resided in Scotland in the eighteenth century and wrote several publications on all facets of dentistry. However, his greatest contributions were in tooth replacement. Hunter received his dental training and anatomy through the assistance of "resurrectionists," who were basically grave robbers. Hunter, along with these men, extracted teeth from the unearthed cadavers (bodies) for his studies. He was able to utilize what he learned from the cadavers and applied this knowledge to living human beings. He successfully transplanted teeth from one human to another. This procedure, however, was not pursued due to two significant factors. First, there was the risk of the spread of disease in transferring a tooth from one person to another. Secondly, at this time it was becoming quite fashionable to wear false teeth. Although Hunter's methods may have been unorthodox, the study of dentistry made several advances during his time.

Dental practitioners migrated to the American colonies in the 1700s and devoted themselves primarily to the removal of diseased teeth and insertion of artificial dentures. A major contribution from the dental profession to the future of health care occurred in 1844 when Dr. Horace Wells, a Connecticut dentist, observed an exhibition of people reacting to inhalation of nitrous oxide (laughing gas). He initiated the use of nitrous oxide inhalation during dental therapy and founded the concept of inhalation analgesia and anesthesia. The medical community later modified and adopted inhalation anesthesia as a standard surgical management procedure.

Paul Revere, historically noted for his "midnight ride," was by trade a metalworker who constructed dentures from ivory and gold. George Washington had dentures made of metal and carved ivory, or metal and carved cow teeth, but none made of wood. Until the mid-1800s, dentures continued to be individually constructed by skilled artisans. Gold, silver, and ivory were common components, causing them to be very expensive and available only to the very wealthy. In 1851 a process to harden the juices of certain tropical plants into vulcanized rubber was discovered. The ability to mold this new material against a model of the patient's mouth and attach artificial porcelain teeth allowed the manufacture of less expensive dentures. Later, acrylic plastics replaced the use of rubber and porcelain in denture construction.

John Baker was a professional dentist who came to colonial America from Ireland in the late 1760s. He was one of the first accomplished dentists to migrate to America. He was well known in Boston, Massachusetts, where he maintained his dental practice for many years. One of his pupils in Boston was Paul Revere. Baker worked extensively at building his dental practice. He traveled from Boston to New York and Philadelphia. He also utilized the newspaper to market himself. He is credited with the technique of using gold to fill teeth. At the time of his death, John Baker had attained his goal of becoming a prominent dentist. His practice was well known, as he provided care for several distinguished citizens, including first American president George Washington.

Greene Vardiman Black (1831-1915) was the leading reformer of American dentistry. Black learned his dental skills from his brother, a medical surgeon, and from several prominent dentists in the late 1800s.

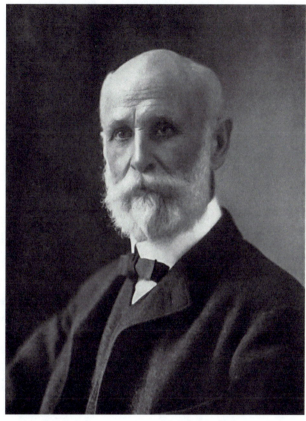

He perfected his skills and progressed rapidly in his practice. Black is best known for his advancements in organized dentistry. Black devised a foot engine that allowed the dentist to keep both hands free while powering the dental drill. He developed modem techniques for filling teeth based upon biological principles and microscopic evaluation. Black also noted a densely matted bacterial coating on the teeth, and he proposed that dental caries and periodontal diseases were infections initiated by Bacteria. It was not until the early 1960s, however, that scientific evidence confirmed this theory. He shared his achievements through his teachings at schools throughout Illinois, his home state. Eventually, he became the dean of Northwestern University Dental School. He was also a professor of operative dentistry and oral pathology. Black performed most of his research at the university. He utilized a method of microscopically sectioning teeth to describe the physical properties of enamel. He was able to use this knowledge to standardize cavity preparation of teeth. Black used the information he collected in his research to become the first to teach students about an idea called "extension for preservation." This idea is integral to cavity preparation. This is a basic concept which is still utilized in dentistry today. Black is also noted for his development of a standardization of dental terminology, instruments, and amalgam-filling materials. Much of today's modern dentistry is based on the research of Black. One of Black's main accomplishments was the development of the five cavity classifications that are still in use today.

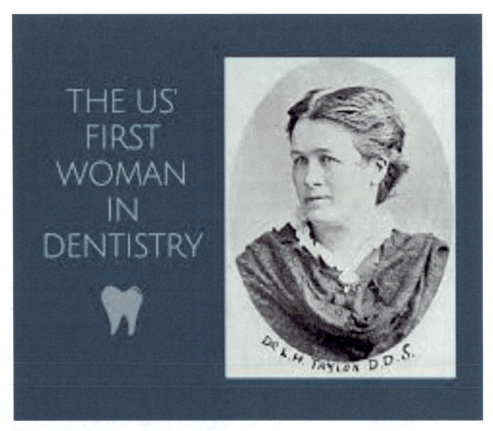

Lucy Hobbs Taylor is distinguished as being the first woman to graduate from an accredited dental school. She earned her degree from the Ohio College of Dental Surgery. She began her dental career in the mid-1860s and continued her practice for over fifty years in the eastern portion of the United States.

C. Edmund Kells was a dental pioneer who lived in the late 1890s. He performed experiments in many dental techniques and conveniences, which are still used today. He was the first dentist to incorporate electricity into his office. This allowed him to use the first electric dental drill that was developed by the S. S. White Company. In addition to his advancements in dental instruments, Kells is noted for being the first dentist to employ a dental assistant. He employed women to assist for him at chairside, to mix dental materials, and to maintain treatment notes. Kells's main contribution to dentistry is in the field of dental radiology. Upon hearing of Conrad Roentgen's discoveries in this area, Kells constructed his own x-ray machine. He used his assistants as subjects so that he was able to develop the first known dental x-ray. Interestingly, he accomplished this task just one year after Roentgen's developments. While Kells was quite accomplished in his achievement, he unfortunately did not realize the dangers of x-rays. He eventually developed cancer in his right hand after years of working with his x-ray equipment. He underwent several surgical procedures, but eventually lost his right hand and arm. He continued to lecture on dentistry until the late 1920s when, due to the excruciating pain he experienced from his condition, he committed suicide.

In the 20th century the Dental profession grow at faster speed and the Scientific dental skills, techniques and procedures were introduced to the stage of modern dentistry, when every 15 minutes a new Dental restorative material is introduced for the use by qualified professionals.

The Amalgam War

Amalgam is one of the most basic substances utilized in dentistry. It is a composite of mercury and alloys including silver, tin, nickel, and copper. Mercury is a hazardous substance that must be handled with caution. Amalgam was first introduced by M. Traveau in the mid-1820s. He demonstrated the use of this silver-based paste as a tooth-filling material. However, due to mechanical problems with the necessary setting time and ultimate expansion, it did not gain much popularity among dentists.

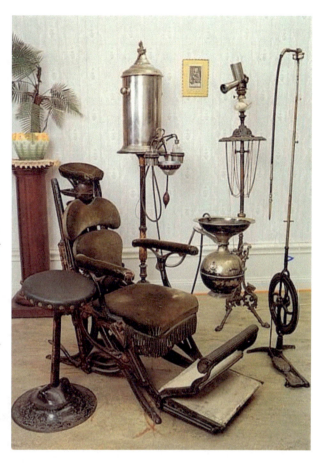

The use of amalgam in the United States is first noted in the early 1830s. The Crawcour brothers introduced amalgam to New York City in 1833, calling it a "royal mineral succedaneum." This title was used since amalgam was hailed as a successor to gold, which was used almost exclusively at that time. Unfortunately, the Crawcours were unethical and unscrupulous. As dentists, they tended to do things that were considered malpractice. A controversy developed regarding their methods that lingered even after they had vacated the dental scene. The "Amalgam War" became so heated that the use of amalgam was considered grounds for malpractice. It wasn't until much later, after amalgam was significantly improved, that its use became acceptable. Even today, you'll hear or read about controversies over the use of mercury in restoration.

Historical background of Dental Surgery Assistant (DSA)

Dr. C. Edmund Kells of New Orleans, USA, hired the first Dental Assistant in 1855. Kells hired a woman as a "Lady in Attendance", so that female patients could respectably come to his office unattended. It was found that these individuals could be enlisted to perform routine dental office chores in the operatory as well as in the business office. Dental assistants continue to serve as office helpers until World War II, when there was a crucial shortage of labour to meet the demand of dental care for military personals. Thus, the Dental Assistants were used in the dental services in the military units, where assistants were trained to work at chair side as an attempt to improve the dental care productivity. Dentists, who trained and worked with the Assistants in the military, retained the concepts of use of auxiliary staff on returning to the civilian practice. So, the concept of involvement of Dental Surgery assistant in actual chair side work came into the existence.

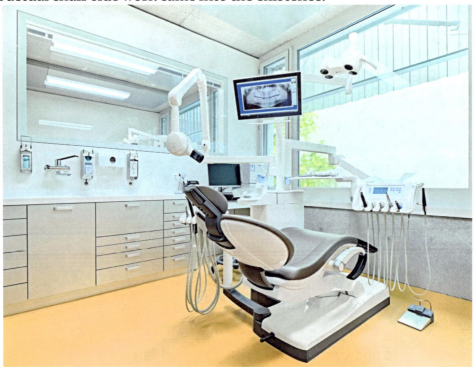

Dental assisting has experienced several significant changes in more recent years. The first major change was in 1960s with the advent of four-handed, sit-down dentistry, which necessitated that a Dental Assistant be actively employed in the delivery of patient care. Operatory design and the use of work simplification principals were introduced to make more efficient working environment, with necessary involvement of the DSA. In 1961 the US government also granted the program to train the dental students to work using the concept of four-handed dentistry. Since then, the profession of the DSA got formal approval to be an important part of the Dental Profession as an auxiliary staff.

The first organization of the Dental Assistants, the Education and Efficiency Society, was formed in 1921 by Juliette Southard in New York City. Other societies also started to form in different cities, and in 1924 the societies met together for the first time on a national level in USA. This organization, the American Dental Assistants' Association (ADAA) remains the recognized professional association of DSA in USA. The ADAA met for the first time in conjunction with the American Dental Association (ADA) in 1924. Since that time, the two organizations, as well as the American Dental Hygienists' Association (ADHA), continue to meet simultaneously at annual sessions.

The need for educational guidance for the DSA was recognized in 1930, when the National Curriculum Committee of the ADAA was formed. In 1937 the Education Committee was introduced which initiated a program to provide official recognition to educationally qualified DSA. Later, the standards of education were standardized for the Certification of the DSA.

The demand and the scope of Dental Assistants in the field of Dentistry have increased many folds in the last few decades.

CHAPTER 2
THE DENTAL OFFICE

The dental office is composed of several different areas, each of which has its own function. The following offers a brief description of each area of the office. Keep in mind that dental offices may vary in their makeup.

THE RECEPTION AREA

The design of the reception area of a dental office is very important as this area gives a patient his or her first impression of the office. Therefore, it is important that the room be set up and decorated with this concept in mind. The reception area is where the patient waits for the appointment with the dentist. The decor of the area should be relaxed and comfortable. Soft lighting and music will help the patient relax while waiting. Also, current, and various kinds of periodicals help to make the waiting time less stressful. The reception area should contain some comfortable chairs for patients who are waiting. There should be some attractive pictures on the walls. Current magazines that appeal to a variety of interests should be available for the patients' reading. If the dentist works with quite a few children, there should be an area with a few quiet toys and books to keep them entertained while they wait. Noisy toys would be out of place in an office setting. Some dentists have an aquarium of tropical fish in the waiting area. Watching the fish has a calming effect on children or other patients who have a fear of visiting the dentist. Keep the reception area at a comfortable temperature. A carelessly kept reception room suggests to clients that the dentist will be careless, too.

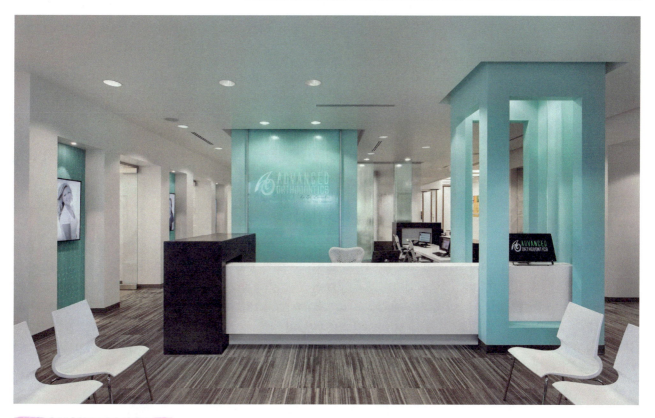

THE BUSINESS AREA

The business area is the "nerve center" of any dental office. It can be broken down into several "subareas."

The reception area:

The reception area is where patients are greeted upon arrival. This is also the area where patient appointments are made and confirmed either in person or via telephone by the receptionist.

The Billing and collection area:

It is in this area that payment by the patients made and all the money are collected. The billing or all related forms, like of insurance claim, etc., are completed in this area. Sometimes their duties are completed at the reception or payment desk. Payments are also collected, or bills sent (sometimes other financial arrangements are made) from this section of the office. Basically, this department is for all billing submitted and payments received, thus making it one of the most important departments for the maintenance of the office.

Office expenses:

This department handles all payments and expenses of the dental office. It's here that the maintenance of payroll, bill payment, and all other office expenses are kept. The term "office overhead" is used to describe all the expenses required to run the office. The business manager can determine the profit of the office by subtracting the total office expenses from the total revenue received.

THE OPERATORY

The operatory, sometimes called the treatment room, is the heart of the dental office. The operatory is where all dental procedures are completed. Operatories will differ from office to office depending on the needs and preferences of the dentist. For example, the operatory of a general dentist will contain the equipment, tools, and materials necessary to complete a variety of procedures. The operatory of a specialist will be quite different. It will contain only those tools needed to handle the dentist's specialized area of dentistry. You will learn about the different tools needed for dental specialties later.

THE LABORATORY

The dental laboratory is where all auxiliary dental procedures are performed. For example, it is in this department where dental models are made or fabricated. Dental laboratories are different in all offices. Some dentists perform quite a bit of their own lab work or they may even employ a lab technician and, therefore, require a larger lab area. Other dentists maintain a smaller laboratory, as their in-house lab work is limited. In some dental offices, the laboratory work is sent to outside laboratories. However, wherever the lab work is accomplished, the dental laboratory is an important part of the dental practice.

THE STERILIZATION AREA

The sterilization area in a dental office is that place where all the dental instruments are cleaned and sterilized. The stringent regulations for dental offices with regard to the operation of this area, are important for anyone responsible for the cleaning and sterilization of instruments.

The sterilization area is divided into three smaller areas—the contaminated area, the sterilized area, and the storage area. Any dental instrument, used during a patient procedure, is first placed in the contaminated area. Here, they are cleaned and disinfected. Once this process is complete, the instruments are ready for the sterilizing area. There are several types of equipment which can be found in the sterilization area, such as an autoclave, cold sterilization solution, a chemiclave, or any combination of these. Once the instruments go through the sterilization process, they are put into the storage area in their sterilized containers and are so kept until they are used again.

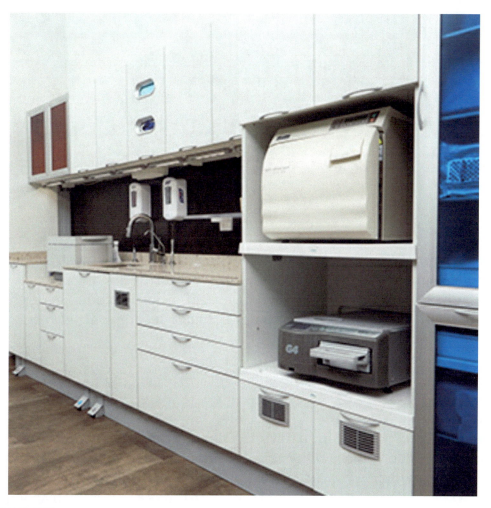

THE DARKROOM

Dental x-rays are developed in a darkroom. A darkroom is a small room which is "light-tight" and specifically designed for x-ray development. A dentist may have an automatic developing machine or may complete this procedure manually. In either case, the x-ray is a vital diagnostic tool for the dentist and proper developing techniques must be always utilized. The darkroom, therefore, must be designed and maintained efficiently for the use of the dentist.

CHAPTER 3

THE DENTAL HEALTH TEAM

Several team members are required to help to make a dental office operation smooth, with adequate efficiency. A member of the dental team must be physically and mentally healthy. The scope of the duties of a dental office staff requires a person who can handle a crisis, work well with different types of people, become a team player on the dental health team, and be willing to grow professionally. The must also be neat, reliable, well organized, and well oriented.

The various important components of the dental team are as follows:

The Dentist

The dentist is the most important part of the dental team. He or she is the center of the dental office. The main responsibility of the dentist is to perform or directly oversee all dental procedures performed in the office. The dentist is ultimately responsible for every aspect of the office. At one time or another the dentist may be faced with an emergency. He or she must be able to act in a responsible manner and strive to maintain a calm atmosphere in the office. Anyone whose goal it is to practice dentistry quickly realizes the rigorous educational background required to earn such a degree.

The prospective dentist must first complete a five-to-six-year graduate college program. The dental school program generally involves five years of intense study and learning, followed by one-year clinical attachments. Dentists in most of the countries usually must pass similar boards. The new dentist, after completing the required education and training and passing the license eligibility requirements of the state or country in which he or she will practice, is qualified to perform the duties of general dentistry. These functions may include procedures such as cleanings, fillings, extractions, root canals, dentures, and bridges. The general dentist who desires to expand on these functions may do so with continued education. A minimum of an additional 2-3 years of education and training is necessary for a dentist to specialize in a particular field of dentistry. Some examples of dental specialists are endodontists, orthodontists, periodontists, and so on.

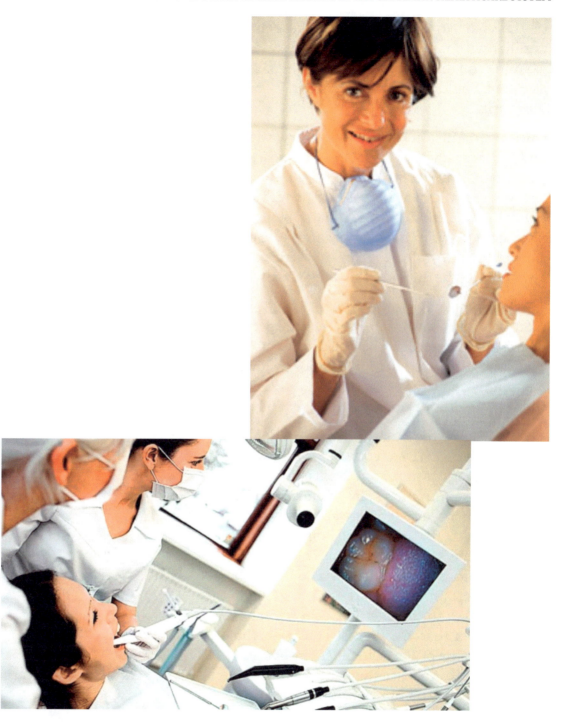

The Dental Assistant

The dental assistant is also an important part of the dental team. The assistant acts as the dentist's "right hand" as he or she directly aids the dentist in performing various procedures. The assistant's responsibilities include preparing the examination room for a procedure to be performed. He or she would then greet and seat the patient comfortably in the chair in preparation for the dentist's arrival. A dental assistant must also be familiar with radiographic procedures and in many countries first need to pass a radiology examination in order to take dental x-rays (HARP Certification). In this capacity, the assistant could take emergency x-rays or even a complete series of x-rays for dental diagnosis.

Once the dentist enters the operatory, the dental assistant should have the instruments and x-rays ready for the doctor. The assistant will then sit chairside with the doctor and participate in performing "four-handed dentistry." (Four-handed dentistry is described this way because the dentist uses two hands plus the assistant's two hands—these equals four hands). The chairside duties that a dental assistant may perform depend on the dental practice act laws of the country and state or province in which the dental office is located. Though in many of the Asian and African countries, there is still no clear-cut practice act law defining the duties of the Dental Assistants.

The assistant may also be responsible for handing the dentist whatever instruments and materials he or she may need. Once the patient is dismissed, the dental assistant will clean, disinfect, and sterilize the operatory and instruments according to regulated standards. These are of the utmost importance in protecting those involved from disease and cross-contamination (transmission of disease from one person to another). The assistant would then prepare the operatory for the next patient.

The education required to become a dental assistant varies from country to country. Dental Surgery Assistant program is generally of 2-years duration in Canada. The qualifications necessary were acquired in the past mainly through hands-on training. Basically, the assistant learned his or her responsibilities and duties via on-the-job training. Certainly, there are advantages and disadvantages to this method. One foremost advantage is that the dentist can train the assistant to his or her own office's needs and philosophies. Another advantage for the assistant is that he or she will be earning a salary while being trained for a position. The overshadowing disadvantage, however, is in the shortcoming of education. The dental assistant in this scenario will learn techniques used by a particular dentist and dental office. If, in the future, the assistant is

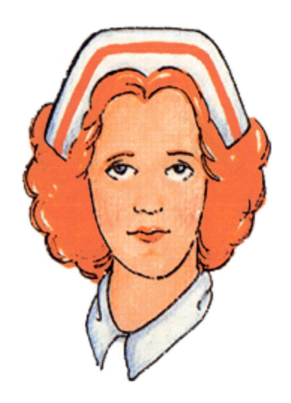

interested in working for another dental office, the lack of a well-rounded education will prohibit him or her from being able to change jobs easily in the workforce. A training program can prepare DSA to become part of the dental team to work more effectively, and to become invaluable to the dentist when performing chairside procedures. The assistant aids the dentist in completing procedures more quickly and efficiently, thus aiding in the comfort of the patient. The dental assistant is also the primary user of the sterilization and infection-control practices that will be discussed in detail later in the other chapters. In some offices, the dental assistant must function in many capacities. The dental office in which he or she works may not employ a business manager, receptionist, or other members of a dental team. In such offices, the dental assistant assumes the front office duties of a receptionist and business manager. You will learn more about these duties and job possibilities as you read on.

The Dental Hygienist

Another important member of a good and efficient Dental Team is Dental Hygienist. Most dental hygienists work in private dental offices. Some also work in hospitals, nursing homes and public health clinics. Some dental hygienists with advanced education and experience may teach in dental schools and dental hygiene education programs. There are also opportunities in research, office management, business administration and companies providing dental-related materials and equipment.

The main responsibilities of the dental hygienist are in providing dental care and in educating the patient in preventive dentistry. Some of the hygienist's functions may include taking x-rays, preparing models of teeth for diagnosis, recording case histories and chart conditions of the oral cavity, polishing restorations (cavity preparations), and applying fluoride treatments.

The major duties of the dental hygienist are to prepare the patient for the necessary procedures and clean the patient's teeth. It is at these times that the patient is educated on the importance of daily oral care and preventive dentistry. The hygienist is also concerned with gingiva maintenance for the patient. The hygienist will treat dental patients every four to six months. The hygienist is responsible for maintaining this time schedule. The function of the hygienist is to prepare the oral cavity of the patient so that the dentist can easily assess and diagnose the oral condition. The education requirements for the dental hygienist are significantly more stringent than that of the dental assistant. The prospective hygienist is required to complete a minimum of two years of training within an accredited dental hygiene program. Upon completion of such a program, the graduate must pass required written and clinical exams to function as Dental Hygienist.

The registered hygienist may perform a variety of duties, including performing cleanings, preparing models, and taking x-rays. He or she is governed by the dental practice act of the state or province in which he or she practices.

Duties of Dental Hygienist:

Dental hygienists perform a wide range of services - primarily in preventative oral health care. Their responsibilities vary according to the specific regulations set by each state but generally include the following:

.

- Assessing dental condition and needs of patient; using patient screening procedures, to include medical history review, dental charting, and perio charting; taking patient vital signs as required. Examining teeth and gums as well as inspecting the neck and head to identify any abnormalities or potential health problems
- Removing calculus, stains, and plaque (hard and soft deposits) from all surfaces of the teeth
- Developing and implementing individualized dental care plans for patients
- Applying preventative materials, such as sealants and fluorides, to the teeth
- Taking and developing dental x-rays
- Teaching patients about good oral hygiene and nutrition
- Making molds of patients' teeth used for evaluating treatment
- discharge planning, and patient/family teaching under the supervision of a qualified dentist
- Providing chair-side assistance to dentist in the performance of special tests, procedures, and complex treatments.
- Assists with or institutes emergency measures for sudden adverse developments during treatment of patients.
- Performs patient triage and initiates patient care as appropriate for walk-in patients.
- Assists in preparation of patient care areas, and in the patient admission, transfer, and discharge process, as required
- prepares reports and assists, as required, with patient reception, telephone calls, routine triage, and other office duties.

In some countries, their roles have expanded to include:

- Placing and removing filling materials, temporary fillings and periodontal dressings
- Smoothing and polishing metal restorations
- Preparing clinical and laboratory diagnostic tests for the dentist to interpret
- Administering anesthetics

The Receptionist / Front-Desk Dental Office Administrators (DOA)

The receptionist / DOA in a dental office is a very important person, as he or she makes the first impression on the dentist's patients. It is crucial, for this reason, that the dentist employ a person who is courteous and friendly. The Front-Desk administrator is the dentist's link to his or her patients. If a patient is uncomfortable or feels that a front-desk staff is not helpful, the dentist stands the risk of the patient going to another office. The reception is, in a sense, the "hub" of the office. It is the responsibility of receptionist / DOA to maintain the flow of the office. A good receptionist / DOA possesses excellent communication skills and can talk easily with the patients. Organization is another invaluable skill of the receptionist / DOA. It is his or her duty, for example, to schedule patients' visits in a manner that is convenient for both patients and the doctor. Finally, the receptionist / DOA must be able to maintain records on each patient regarding billing and insurance information. A typical day for a receptionist / DOA includes the performance of a multitude of various tasks. He or she must be prepared to greet each patient who enters the office. If a patient is new, it is the responsibility of the receptionist / DOA to collect information such as a health history, personal information, and insurance/billing information. As each patient concludes a visit with the dentist, the receptionist / DOA schedules follow-up visits and completes all billing inquiries. It is easy to understand why the receptionist / DOA can be considered as one of the main driving forces of the office because it's his or her responsibility to keep the office running smoothly. The trained and educated Dental Office Administrators are always an asset for a dental office. The Administrators should have excellent communication and organizational skills. The receptionist / DOA/administrator needs to be people-oriented because he or she is the first impression the patient receives of the dentist. A good receptionist / DOA can easily be one of a dentist's greatest assets in the office. Some receptionists / DOAs perform duties that include the receipt of money and the banking of the dental office; however, it is generally handled by the Office Administrators or Office Managers.

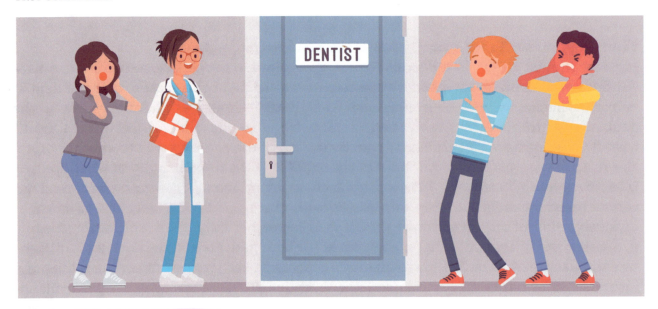

THE RECEPTIONIST / DOA'S DUTIES

Reception is an opportunity to establish a positive relationship with patients. Receptionist / DOA, who is enthusiastic about his or her work will help make the dental office a more relaxed setting and more enjoyable for patients and other employees. The receptionist / DOA in the Dental Office must be flexible enough to accommodate the unexpected. Any number of events might change the pace of the day, so carefully scheduled. A seemingly routine appointment might turn out to be a complicated and time-consuming procedure. An emergency may arise that must be scheduled in immediately. Throughout the sometimes-chaotic changes in the appointment schedule, one must remain calm and cheerful to greet patients and soothe those in distress. In short, the receptionist / DOA is responsible for creating and maintaining a good social, physical, and professional atmosphere in the dental office. There are four key words that describe the ideal performance of a receptionist / DOA. They are promptly, pleasantly, properly, and politely.

Greeting Patients

It is very important on the part of receptionist / DOA to have pleasing telephone and personal communication skills to create a favorable impression for the Dental Office. It is the duty of the receptionist / DOA to greet and welcome the patient to the dental office on his or her visit. The very first thing to do when a patient arrives is to acknowledge him or her. Patients appreciate a personal touch, which can make them feel more important as individuals.

First Impressions

It is significant that all the Dental Office staff wear the clothes that are clean, neat, and in good condition, with professional taste. Although the receptionist / DOA and other business assistants normally do not wear uniforms, the dental assistant and hygienist usually do wear a light-colored smock over white uniform pants and white shoes. When the receptionist / DOA is also the dental assistant, he or she normally wears a uniform. The care one takes in presenting a clean, neat, efficient appearance will go a long way with clients who already feel nervous about their dental appointment.

The Business Manager

The business manager of a dental office represents the financial aspects of the office. It is the responsibility of this person to maintain all the financial records of the office. Certainly, the person who holds this position must be someone whom the dentist can trust explicitly. The business manager has access to all the data of the office with regard to collected income and outstanding debts. The manager's job duties include making collections, ensuring the payment of bills

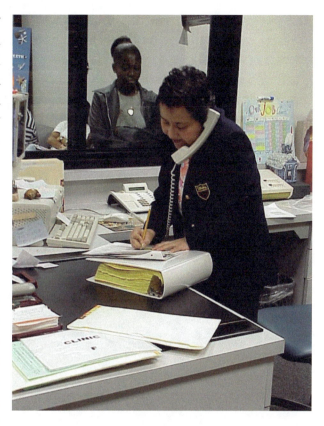

incurred, and the preparing staff payroll. The duties of the business manager do not end with money collected and spent in the office. He or she may also be involved in projections for the office. For example, the manager may oversee watching the production of the office and looking for new means of marketing the business to improve the "bottom line," also known as the profit. If a business fails to earn a profit, it is difficult for the dentist to continue his or her practice. Maintaining inventory is another task for which the manager may be responsible. He or she may oversee maintaining the stock of both dental and office supplies for the business. The position of business manager does not necessarily require a formal education. However, it would be wise for the dentist to employ a manager who holds a background in basic accounting skills. The manager must also possess excellent business and organizational skills. He or she must be able to recognize whether an office is profitable or struggling and how to correct any problems. A manager who has a sincere interest in the office will certainly be an asset to the dentist and will be able to run the office efficiently and effectively. Remember that the Dental Assistant of the Dental Hygienist may be the person who also perform the duties of the business manager and receptionist / DOA in small dental offices.

The Laboratory Technician

The laboratory technician is actually the craftsperson of the dental office. The technician is the person who fabricates the prosthetic (replacement) devices, which the dentist prepares for the patients. The devices he or she makes can range from full or partial dentures to crowns, veneers, or any other custom-fitted dental prosthesis. Once an impression of a patient's mouth is taken, it is sent to the technician with the dentist's prescription for final production. The dentist's prescription is written with very specific instructions as to fit and style. It is the skill and capability of the technician that aids in creating the final prosthesis. In many countries its illegal for a technician to prepare any prosthesis without a dentist's prescription.

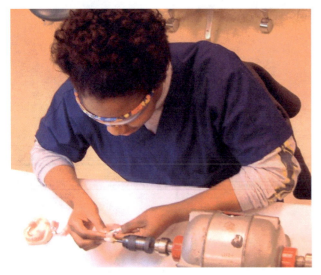

The process by which the lab work is done is one that requires patience and a certain dexterity. Educational programs are available where one can be trained as a lab technician. Many assistant technicians also learn from on-the-job training. However, a qualified lab technician is an asset to any dental office. The work a technician does is very precise and can sometimes be complicated. It is essential that a technician provide quality and timely work for the dentist so that the goal of having a patient who is comfortable and satisfied, is met. This goal can be accomplished only if the technician is conscientious and maintains good communication with the dentist. Anyone with such tools can certainly have a rewarding career in this field.

CHAPTER 4

WORKING CONDITIONS IN DIFFERENT CLINICAL ENVIRONMENTS

A broad range of career opportunities is available for the dental assistant, dental hygienist, dental technician, dental office administrators, and other auxiliary staff in modern day dentistry. They become an integral part of the dental team in a variety of settings. Broadly, in addition to the opportunities in the Hospitals, we can divide the modern dental offices in the following categories, in which the various dental auxiliaries or commonly known as assistants can become a team member.

General Office

There can be two types of general dental offices: a private office and a group practice.

Private office. This type of office usually consists of one general dentist with an auxiliary staff (members of the dental team). In such a setting the dental assistant is responsible for providing assistance to the dentist in preventive and restorative dental procedures.

Group practice. A group practice is formed when one or more partners make up the dental office. Often, the partners will also include one or more associates in the practice. The dental assistant, dental hygienist, dental office administrators, or dental technician working in this setting must attuned to the different working practices of each dentist. It is their function to fit into the dentist's mode of work in order to provide the necessary assistance. Each dentist will have his or her own techniques when working and the dental auxiliaries must be aware of these in order to perform their duties effectively. It is important to remember that the goal is to provide the best possible care to the patient and the dental auxiliaries plays a major role in attaining this goal.

Endodontic Office

A dentist in an endodontic office is a specialist who deals primarily with teeth that develop a type of infection. The major procedures performed in this office are root canals and their related functions. The role of the dental assistant in this office is unique. The assistant not only provides assistance to the dentist, but also must possess good patient management skills. Most of the patients entering the endodontic office are experiencing some form of dental discomfort. In addition, they may be anxious because their problem requires the expertise of a specialist. It is the expectation of the dentist that the assistant will be able to provide some assurance to the patient upon entering the *operatory* (sometimes called the treatment room).

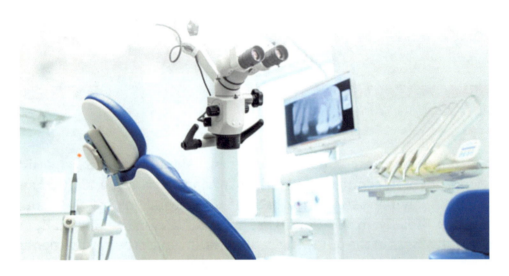

Pediatric (Pedodontic) Dental Office

The dental assistant working in a pediatric (sometimes called pedodontic) dental office will assist with the treatment of children aged 2–13, although older teenagers and young adults may also be seen. The assistant in this setting works with a unique patient group. It's necessary for the assistant to be able to feel comfortable in this office as the young patient often requires a different style of management. To operate in a pediatric dental office the assistant must be prepared to handle a child who may be frightened, crying, or difficult to manage. The young patient may not be cooperative about the procedure to be done and it is at this time that the assistant must refer to his or her management skills to effectively assist the dentist.

Periodontic Office

The periodontist is a specialist who is concerned with the supporting tissues of the teeth. This involves treatment of the gums, the *palate* (the roof of the mouth), and all oral *mucosa* (mucous membranes) and soft tissues. The patient referred to the periodontic office would require preventive dental work as well as some surgical procedures. The dental assistant must be aware of periodontal gum disease and its treatments in order to provide effective aid to the dentist.

Prosthodontic Office

The patient who requires the prosthetic replacement of missing teeth would be referred to a prosthodontist. The specialist in this office would treat the patient with an array of prosthetic devices including a removable full or partial denture, crowns, bridges, or dental implants. This can be a unique and interesting office in which the dental assistant is a very important part of the dental team. Once again, the assistant must be aware of the special needs of the patients in order to effectively aid the dentist.

Orthodontic Office

The specialist in the orthodontic office is concerned with the correction of *malocclusion* (teeth that do not come together properly), which calls for the straightening of teeth for cosmetic and functional purposes. The patient group in this type of office was, at one time, mainly made up of adolescents. However, in recent times, more and more adults are seeking the assistance of the orthodontist for both cosmetic and functional treatment. Therefore, the dental assistant in this office must be prepared to work with both young and adult patients and assist in meeting the needs of each.

Oral Surgery Office

The dental assistant working in an oral surgeon's office would assist the dentist in the treatment of *oral pathology* (the study of diseases of the mouth). The oral surgeon is concerned with a wide range of dental procedures including extractions, the reduction of fractures, the diagnosis of tumors, and other oral pathologies. While it can be a more intense setting for the dental assistant, it's nonetheless interesting and the assistant's role is vital.

Other Office Locations

Hospital Setting

A dentist may treat a patient who is currently receiving care in a hospital. This may appear to be an unusual setting for a dentist to see a patient. However, this type of visit can be critical for a patient as he or she is usually in need of emergency treatment. If a hospital patient is experiencing some oral infection or acute trauma, it can interfere with the medical treatment being received. While the hospital setting is unique, it can also provide a very challenging career opportunity for the dentist and dental assistants.

Rural Health Setting

Rural health clinics are generally operated by some government agency. Dental care, in such a setting, consists of two facets—preventive dentistry and clinical care. The role of the dental assistant in such a clinic is mainly to provide chairside aid (help to the dentist during procedures). However, another responsibility of the assistant is to provide education to patients in regard to the promotion of good oral hygiene and the practice of preventive dentistry.

CHAPTER 5

DELEGATION OF DUTIES OF AUXILIARY STAFF IN DENTAL OFFICE

Duties and Settings

According to the Dental auxiliary staff regulation the dentists using the services of dental auxiliaries must post, in a common area of the office, a note that explains duties and functions deemed to be delegated within stipulated settings and/or circumstances. The notice should be readily accessible to all office personnel. Posting this notice, however, is not the end of the dentist's responsibility for adequate supervision of auxiliaries. The Dental Practice Act requires supervision of auxiliaries for all delegated duties.

Delegation of duties and responsibility by the supervising dentist beyond the auxiliary's scope of practice is not only illegal, but also unethical for the dentist and dangerous for his/her patients.

Dentists must also understand that they cannot avoid responsibility for acts committed by auxiliaries under their supervision. Failure to supervise auxiliaries properly can result in Dental Council / State Board disciplinary action against a dentist's license or create a civil lawsuit. As defined in the Dental Practice Act, a *Direct Supervision* means supervision of dental procedures based on instructions given by a licensed dentist who must be physically present in the treatment facility during performance of these procedures. A *General Supervision* means supervision of dental procedures based on instruction given by licensed dentist, but not requiring the physical presence of the supervising dentist during the performance of those procedures.

In dental offices, there are three valuable members of the care-giving team: the dentist, the dental hygienist, and the dental assistant.

DENTAL ASSISTANT

DUTIES AND SETTINGS

In modern day dentistry the dentists are generally hire more assistants to perform routine tasks so that they may devote their own time to more profitable procedures. Most assistants learn their skills on the job, although an increasing number are trained in dental-assisting programs; most programs take 1 year or less to complete. Because of the nature of their work, Dental assistants generally work in a well-lighted, clean environment. Their work area usually is near the dental chair so that they can arrange instruments, materials, and medication and hand them to the dentist when needed. Dental assistants must wear gloves, masks, eyewear, and protective clothing to protect themselves and their patients from infectious diseases. Following safety procedures also minimizes the risks associated with the use of x-ray machines.

Dental assistants perform a variety of patient care, office, and laboratory duties. They work chairside as dentists examine and treat patients. They make patients as comfortable as possible in the dental chair, prepare them for treatment, and obtain their dental records. Assistants hand instruments and materials to dentists and keep patients' mouths dry and clear by using suction or other devices. Assistants also sterilize and disinfect instruments and equipment, prepare trays of instruments for dental procedures, and instruct patients on postoperative and general oral health care.

Some dental assistants prepare materials for impressions and restorations, take dental x rays, and process x-ray film as directed by a dentist. They also may remove sutures, apply topical anesthetics to gums or cavity-preventive agents to teeth, remove excess cement used in the filling process, and place rubber dams on the teeth to isolate them for individual treatment.

Those with laboratory duties make casts of the teeth and mouth from impressions, clean and polish removable appliances, and make temporary crowns. Dental assistants with office duties schedule and confirm appointments, receive patients, keep treatment records, send bills, receive payments, and order dental supplies and materials.

Dental assistants should not be confused with dental hygienists, who are licensed to perform different clinical tasks. In a Dental Office generally following guidelines are followed while delegating the duties to the DSA:

(a) Unless specifically so provided by regulation, a dental assistant may **NOT** perform the following functions or any other activity which represents the practice of dentistry or requires the knowledge, skill, and training of a licensed dentist:
1) Diagnosis and treatment planning; 2) Surgical or cutting procedures on hard or soft tissue; 3) Fitting and adjusting of correctional and prosthodontic appliances; 4) Prescription of medicines; 5) Placement, condensation, carving or removal of permanent restorations, including final cementation procedures; 6) Irrigation and medication of canals, try-in cones, reaming, filing or filling of root canals; 7) Taking of impressions for prosthodontic appliances, bridges or any other structures which may be worn in the mouth; 8) Administration of injectable and/or general anesthesia; 9) Oral prophylaxis procedures.

(b) A dental assistant may perform such basic supportive dental procedures as the following under the *general supervision* of a licensed dentist: 1) Extra-oral duties or functions specified by the supervising dentist; 2) Operation of dental radiographic equipment for the purpose

of oral radiography if the dental assistant has completed the required training of radiology;
3) Examine orthodontic appliances.

(c) A dental assistant may perform such basic supportive dental procedures as the following under the *direct supervision* of a licensed dentist when done so pursuant to the order, control, and full professional responsibility of the supervising dentist. Such procedures shall be checked and approved by the supervising dentist prior to dismissal of the patient from the office of said dentist.

1) Take impressions for diagnostic and opposing models, bleaching trays, temporary crowns and bridges, and sports guards;

2) Apply non-aerosol and non-caustic topical agents;

3) Remove post-extraction and periodontal dressings;

4) Placement of elastic orthodontic separators;

5) Remove orthodontic separators;

6) Assist in the administration of nitrous oxide analgesia or sedation however, a dental assistant shall not start the administration of the gases and shall not adjust the flow of the gases unless instructed to do so by the dentist who shall be present at the patient's chairside at the implementation of these instructions. This regulation shall not be constructed to prevent any person from taking appropriate action in the event of a medical emergency;

7) Hold anterior matrices;

8) Remove sutures;

9) Take intra-oral measurements for orthodontic procedures;

10) Seat adjusted retainers or headgears, including appropriate instructions;

11) Check for loose bands;

12) Remove arch wires;

13) Remove ligature ties;

14) Apply topical fluoride, after scaling and polishing by the supervising dentist or a registered dental hygienist;

15) Place and remove rubber dams;

16) Place, wedge and remove matrices;

17) Cure restorative or orthodontic materials in operative site with light-curing device.

DENTAL HYGIENIST

DUTIES AND SETTINGS

With the support of the hygienist, dentists can provide better professional care to more patients, thus increasing both the quality of the dental treatment and the productivity of the office.

A registered dental hygienist may perform all duties assigned to registered dental assistants, under the supervision of a licensed dentist as specified earlier. However, Dental hygienist may perform the following duties in addition to those mentioned earlier for Dental Surgery Assistant (DSA):

1. Root planning.
2. 2) Polish and contour restorations.
3. Oral exfoliative cytology.
4. Apply pit and fissure sealants.
5. Preliminary examination, including but not limited to: A) Periodontal charting; B) Intra and extra-oral examination of soft tissue; C) Charting of lesions, existing restorations, and missing teeth; D) Classifying occlusion; E) Myofunctional evaluation.
6. The following direct supervision duties of dental assistants:
   - (i)   Taking impressions for diagnostic and opposing models,
   - (ii)   Applying non-aerosol and non-caustic topical agents.
   - (iii)   Removing post-extraction and periodontal dressings.
   - (iv)   Removing sutures.
   - (v)   Taking intra-oral measurements for orthodontic procedures.
   - (vi)   Checking for loose bands.
   - (vii)   Removing ligature ties.
   - (viii)   Applying topical fluoride.
   - (ix)   Placing elastic separators.

7. The following direct supervision duties of registered dental assistants:
   - (i)   Test pulp vitality.
   - (ii)   Removing excess cement from supragingival surfaces of teeth.
   - (iii)   Sizing stainless steel crowns, temporary crowns and bands.
   - (iv)   Temporary cementation and removal of temporary crowns and removal of orthodontic bands.
   - (v)   Placing post-extraction and periodontal dressings.

A registered dental hygienist may perform the procedures set forth below under the *direct supervision* of a licensed dentist when done so pursuant to the order, control and full professional responsibility of the supervising dentist. Such procedures shall be checked and approved by the supervising dentist prior to dismissal of the patient from the office of said dentist:

1) All duties so assigned to a dental assistant or a registered dental assistant, unless otherwise indicated.
2) Periodontal soft tissue curettage.
3) Administration of local anesthetic agents, infiltration and conductive, limited to the oral cavity.
4) Administration of nitrous oxide and oxygen when used as an analgesic, utilizing fail-safe type machines containing no other general anesthetic agents.

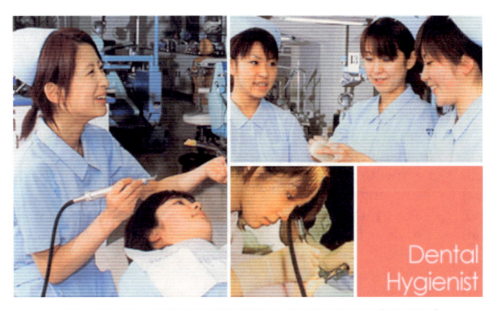

REGISTERED DENTAL HYGIENIST IN EXTENDED FUNCTIONS (RDHEF) DUTIES AND SETTINGS

An RDHEF may perform all duties assigned to dental assistants, registered dental assistants, and registered dental hygienists. In addition to it the RDHEF can also perform the certain specified duties in a Dental Office. An RDHEF may perform the procedures set forth below under the *direct supervision* of a licensed dentist when done so pursuant to the order, control, and full professional responsibility of the supervising dentist. Such procedures shall be checked and approved by the supervising dentist prior to dismissal of the patient from the office of said dentist.

(1) Cord retraction of gingivae for impression procedures.
(2) Take impressions for cast restorations.

(3) Take impressions for space maintainers, orthodontic appliances and guards.
(4) Prepare enamel by etching for bonding.
(5) Formulate indirect patterns for endodontic post and core castings.
(6) Fit trial endodontic filling points.
(7) Apply etchant for bonding restorative materials.

The Dental councils or dental boards in most of the countries require the dentist to examine and diagnose all new patients prior to delegating general supervision duties to auxiliaries.

CHAPTER 6
TEAM MANAGEMENT IN THE DENTAL PRACTICE

The practice of Dentistry has changed dramatically during the past decade. As the number of the persons involved in the dental practice has considerably increased in the modern dentistry, the team effort and its proper management is significant for the efficient delivery of the dental care services. It is a little recognition that goes a long way toward achieving a winning team which benefits everyone.

What is a Team?
The team is a group of independent individuals, usually with different roles and functions, whose combined efforts toward a mutually shared goal are required for the successful completion of a task.

A number of the problems commonly occur, when team functioning is attempted without proper orientation. The following items cover the major reasons for these problems:

1. Absence of clear and shared goals and philosophy
2. Lack of specified decision-making mechanism
3. Use of a decision-making mechanism that attributes more to educational background and professional status than to having the most relevant information
4. Lack of clarity about responsibilities of each team member
5. Closed or any partially open communication channels
6. Absence of a time and method for problem identification, analysis, and solution
7. Insufficient planning time or and inadequate planning process
8. Lack of mechanism for resolving team conflicts
9. Inadequate selection procedures for team members

Unresolved team problems can be extremely costly. Friction among team members can be felt by patients and may result in inadequate care of patients, loss of patients and high cost of the treatment procedure.

Team rapport is needed to keep the dentist in touch with the patients. In a busy practice, auxiliary staff serves as a communication bridge.

Theories of Management:

Underlying assumptions, values, and beliefs are guiding factors in our behaviour, though most of the time they remain unidentified as such. The manner in which someone goes about managing or participating on a team is also determined in large measure by her or his underlying beliefs about people: what motivates them, what they need, and how they function. McGregor described two different theories of management, based on the underlying beliefs about the people. The theories are designated simply as **X and Y theory**.

Theory X's assumption about the average people are the following:
1. They are lazy, preferring to work as little as possible,
2. they dislike responsibility or incapable of handling it,
3. they prefer to be dependent on others, or want to be led by others,
4. they are incapable of self-control, so must be controlled by others,
5. they cannot find satisfaction of important needs in work and must, therefore seek basic satisfaction outside the work setting.

The assumptions that theory Y makes about the people are quite different. They include the following:
1. They prefer to be active rather than passive,
2. they are capable of assuming responsibility and find satisfaction in doing so,
3. they prefer being independent, finding greater satisfaction in not having to look to others for direction,
4. they are capable of finding basic satisfaction and self-fulfillment in their work,
5. they are capable of self-control, not needing control from outside.

The theory X assumptions lead to the team unit or organization having:
(i)   a very clear chain of command, in which the top of the hierarchy both directs and controls the bottom. There is usually little communication up the line, with the result that the person directing does not know the effects of his or her directives.

(ii)   A very narrow task specialization. The assignments are made so that each individual has a small and narrowly defined task that he or she does well. The result is that personnel cannot substitute for each other, even though the tasks are within the scope of their competence. More important, they often do not understand each other's jobs, so that needless conflicts can arise because of lack of knowledge and awareness.

However, on the other hand, the theory Y assumptions lead to the team unit having:
(i)   a very democratic set up, in which the work is distributed in a well-mannered way, making the function smoother and function less. The

members of teamwork like a well-oiled machinery, to achieve the same goal.

(ii)   A combined effort for the same goal. As the members show interest and know each other's work, the conflicts are fewer and temporary replacement of any absent staff member is possible internally only.

Importance of Teamwork in Dental Office:

As many staff members are involved in almost all the modern Dental offices, the proper teamwork is of utmost importance for the smooth and successful functioning. Any rift or ego problem among the staff members at any level can have direct effect on the day-to-day functioning of the Dental office. As mentioned in the McGregor's X and Y theory, the inclusion of the Y theory is essential for long-term benefit and success. The motivated staff members, like in any other organization, can be of great value in a Dental Office. All the staff members should be given their due importance in the setup, as running a Dental Office is a team effort. The mutual respect, irrespective of the education and position held, is a great contributory factor in evolving the individuals to work as a team. It has been generally recognized that they are not unlike the mortar that bonds individual bricks into a wall, or the spokes that make a wheel so strong. They are a really big group, consisting of Dental Hygienists, dental assistants, and Dental Technicians, who are working worldwide to help bind together the team of dental professionals who each day seek to improve the oral health of their patients. Their work is so significant that two decades ago the American Dental Association and American Dental Assistants Association established Dental Assistants Recognition Week. Its purpose is to promote teamwork and recognize dental assistants as an essential part of the dental team. The idea behind establishing this Recognition week was that since they are such a vital part of the dental office, all auxiliary dental staff need to be appreciated for their contribution in the field of dentistry. They help the dentist by performing dental treatment procedures they are licensed to do, thereby maximizing both production and profits

They also help in improving the patient's communication in the alien environment of the Dental Office, as generally patients are often more willing to ask questions and express concerns to someone other than the dentist.

Now a days in a modern Dental Office set up there are many duties delegated to the auxiliary staff that in turn allow dentists to do much more diagnostic and other work. This, and the fact that the qualified Dental Hygienist and Dental Assistants and RDA's are high-quality sorts of individuals, goes a long way in helping to reduce the stress and strain on dentists.

Before introduction of the ultra-high-speed handpiece in the late 1950s, there was less need for direct patient care, but after its introduction, dental assistants became more important, resulting in a tremendous evolution in duties. Due to it the DSA's got more involved with direct patient care, which in turn gave them the opportunity to promote more togetherness in the office because of their direct involvement in the chair side work, which helped to integrate them into the team.

Whether its calming an anxious child or performing one of a myriad of other challenging duties, dental assistants work to enhance the oral health of the society.

Management of Team Effort in Dental Office:

It was not long time back, when Dentists were struggling with the issues of personal management. However, it has been realized in last decade or so that what makes an effective leader and helper, also makes an effective dentist. A Weak Management Skill in a Dentist generally fails to produce a dentist, who is effectively successful in working with patients.

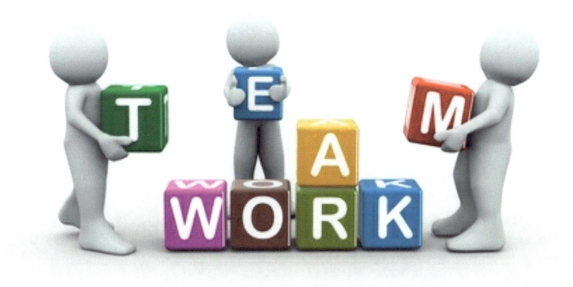

Responsibility Development:

Very little has been written about responsibility development in dentistry, perhaps because dentists have never before been so dependent upon the actions of others for success and mental well-being. However, the past decade has changed all that forever. Preventive dentistry and increased utilization of auxiliary personnel, two significant and irreversible developments, have brought dentistry face to face with its lack of "know how" in getting people to seek and accept increasing amounts of responsibility. Disappointment at "preventive failures" is rampant in the profession, and the stresses associated with more auxiliaries in offices are regular matter of concern among dentists and staffs alike. Stresses among auxiliaries have even been cited as a major cause of failures of group practices.

Some dentists seem naturally able to work efficiently with both auxiliaries and patients. In fact, careful observation of the recent research studies leads to an interesting conclusion. Those dentists that have highly committed and stable staffs are by and large the same dentists who get people to develop more responsible attitudes toward their dental health care. On the other hand, those dentists that complain of the problems of keeping their staff motivated (or who have excessive personnel turn over) usually have a tougher time getting patients to accept quality preventive dentistry, or to remain motivated to eat more sensibly, or to do a consistently better job with home care. Apparently, a dentist's management attitudes toward staff and patients are remarkable similar.

The inferences of the research stress the need for a dentist to look inside himself before trying to make tactical changes in auxiliary or patient management. It has been felt strongly that a dentist understanding of his self-image is important in deciding how to hire, whom to hire, and how to train. As for personnel and patient management, it has been felt that most dentists were simply imitating others within the profession without any serious study or thoughtful personnel growth and development, during the transition period some 15 – 20 years back. However, now the significance of teamwork and the importance of active whole-hearted involvement of each component of the team in a Dental office, has been realized and most of the Dental Offices are observed to be managed by a very cohesive joint team efforts with the Dentist as its guiding leader, and Dental Hygienist, Dental Surgery Assistant and Dental Technician as important partners of the set up.

GAME RULES FOR DENTAL TEAM MEMBERS
• Be sensitive to the people you work with.
• Make adjustments to cooperate with fellow employees.
• Show interest.
• Express appreciation to teammates.
• Be courteous.
• Be open to new ideas and concepts.
• Keep communication lines open between all staff members.
• Be honest with yourself and others.
• Keep the private business revealed to you by your coworkers to yourself.
• Don't spread rumors—if you have a criticism of an employee, take it directly to that person.
• If misunderstandings occur, clear them up immediately.
• Admit your mistakes.
• Accept constructive criticism graciously and with an open mind.

CHAPTER 7
COMMUNICATING IN THE DENTAL OFFICE

COMMUNICATION

In a layman terms the act of either relaying or receiving information in a variety of situations is called communication. In the process of their working, the staff working in the dental office interacts with the patients and with other staff members, handles incoming and outgoing phone calls, and schedule appointments. To work effectively and to be successful, one needs to be skillful in these types of communication.

The most important elements in the communication process are the message, the sender, the receiver, and feedback. The message is an idea or information that must be transferred from one person to another. The sender is the one who originates the message and sends it. The receiver is the one who receives the message that was sent. When the receiver responds to the message and sends some additional information back to the sender, that reply is called feedback. As a result of feedback, the original sender may revise the original idea and decide upon a different course of action. For this reason, it's very important to communicate clearly and concisely to avoid a mistaken interpretation of the message.

There are four important rules for sending a message, which all the dental office staff members should remember when communicating with others:

(1) Know the receiver:
As each receiver has a different background of culture and experience, a good communicator must avoid misunderstandings by adapting the speech to the listener's needs, expectations, and ability to understand.

(2) Speak clearly and concisely:
One need to speak clearly in a professional manner while dealing with patients. It may be e helpful to mirror the speech-speed of the person with whom you are speaking.

(3) Present information on the receiver's level:
Most of the patients have little, if any, knowledge of dental terminology. So, it is of paramount importance for the staff to take care to explain any technical terms that is used during treatment discussion.

(4) Obtain feedback:

Ask questions to understand and gauge the effectiveness of your communication.

VERBAL COMMUNICATION

The auxiliary staff in the dental office use spoken communication far more than the written words. In developing people skills, conversational skills are extremely important. The staff working in Dental Office must be patient and tactful even on days when everything seems to be going wrong. A patient who is in pain may become irritated easily and require special handling to avoid problem areas. A skillful communication can make the difference between a dissatisfied patient and one who understands your concern for his or her welfare. This difference makes a big change in the attitude of the patient.

NON-VERBAL COMMUNICATION

The messages sent back and forth between the speaker and the listener through body language, though of significant importance, are often overlooked in the communication process. Body language consists of nonverbal symbols, emotions, or other uses of the body that convey a non-spoken message.

It is important to know the basic components of body language so that one can understand the meaning of nonverbal signals, which in turn makes him or her more effective in work in the dental office. It is important to interpret the actual message being sent by the patient. His or her body language is more likely to give the true picture than the actual words being used. The tone of the voice, eye contact, body posture, gestures and facial expression also pay an important role in effective communication.

The most obvious positive facial expression is a smile. Be quick to smile when greeting patients. A sincere smile can go a long way toward relieving anxiety of the visiting patient. But be careful not to force a smile. One should not allow the patient to feel that you are faking your hospitality. Be especially careful to smile only at appropriate moments.

GOOD BODY LANGUAGE FOR THE STAFF OF DENTAL OFFICE

- Face the patient and hold your gaze steady.
- Hold your arms at your sides or gently folded.
- Stand straight with legs upright or sit erect with legs together or gently crossed.
- Keep posture erect but not rigid.
- Stay approximately one arm's length away from the patient.
- Always wear professional attire.
- Always practice good hygiene.
- Keep a relaxed, pleasant facial expression or match the expression of the patient.
- Speak in a moderate and clear vocal tone.

DEVELOPING POSITIVE RELATIONSHIPS WITH PATIENTS

To develop a healthy relation with the patients, the dental office staff should possess the positive personality traits, which make it easier to form positive connections. Every staff member must have patience, tact, kindness, courtesy, and empathy.

For a person who works with many different types of people, patience is probably the most important skill to possess. Patients may be reluctant or embarrassed to discuss their fear of visiting the dentist. All the professionals working in the dental office should be capable to make these people more comfortable and need to gently encourage them. Be sure to explain the dental procedures to them so that they will know what to expect. This will help them to cope with their fear.

Tact means doing and saying the right things at the right time. If you are tactful, you maintain good relations with the patients and avoid offense. Often, it is not what is said that creates the problem, but how it is said.

Kindness means being helpful, compassionate, and friendly. Remember that you are on the patient's side. Remember that patients coming into a dentist's office may be in pain or full of dread at the prospect of having a filling or other work done. Be sensitive to their feelings and help them to understand their feelings. Your kindness towards these patients can put them in a more relaxed frame of mind.

Courtesy means putting the needs of other people before your own. It means cooperating, sharing, and giving. You should deal with all patients on a polite, professional, and impartial basis.

Empathy means being able to feel and understand what the other person is feeling. When you give the patient empathetic feedback, you let the patient know that you fully understand his or her concerns.

RESOLUTION OF CONFLICTS

There are many types of conflict and several situations, which one should be familiar with, in order to successfully handle interpersonal relationships with other staff members and patients. The various methods or techniques by which the conflict can be avoided or resolved, are as follows:
(1) Communication to resolve contention
(2) Avoiding condemnation
(3) Analysis and organization to end confusion
(4) Sticking to the facts to resolve confrontation
(5) Courtesy and consideration for others
(6) Communication
(7) The skill of conciliation
(8) Cooperation

MONITORING OF PATIENTS' FEARS

For many of the patients, a visit to the dentist's office is a very scary experience. Some people will make all sorts of excuses to put off the visit even if they realize it's unwise to do so.

Assess patient behavior. The dentist, hygienist, the dental assistant, and the receptionist /

DOA should all be able to identify the fearful patient. Patient's action as well as his words can help to determine whether the patient has fears, which are unexpressed. It makes the handling of the patient, comparatively easier, in order to allay his or her fears.

Fear responses. The patient may appear very nervous and be unable to make eye contact with you as you greet him or her. This will give an indication that one should speak in a very friendly manner and try to put the patient at ease.

Managing a dental fear. The best way to relax the patient and help dispose of the fear is through information. While preparing for the dental procedure, the auxiliary dental staff need to talk with the patient, in a relaxed manner about the procedure. After that the dentist can go into more detail when he or she comes in to see the patient. All these things develop trust and help the patient to relax during the process.

EFFECTIVE TELEPHONE COMMUNICATION IN DENTAL OFFICE

Since the telephone is the main line of communication between the dental office and the patients, anyone who answers the phone or makes calls must develop a pleasing telephone personality.

Phone behavior is an important part of public relations in any office. A truly pleasing telephone personality always pleases fellow employees and the patients. Telephone courtesy and interest in the patient are important parts of keeping patients happy with the dental practice.

Here are some things that one should be sure to do, while receiving and making calls in the dental office:

(1) Answer promptly-
Make sure that there is always someone there to answer the telephone. Try to answer by the second ring and avoid letting it ring more than three times.

(2) Identify yourself-
After greeting the person on the other side of the phone, immediately give the names of the dentist's clinic.

(3) Speak pleasantly-
Speak naturally in a relaxed, low pitch and remember to smile so that your friendly personality comes through in your voice.

(4) Be courteous-
Always use polite language—please, thank you, pardon me—and give your caller your full attention.

(5) Show interest in the caller and their problems

(6) Explain interruptions-

If you must leave the telephone to get information or put the caller on hold to answer another line, explain why and give the caller a chance to respond. Be considerate of the patient's time as well as your own. And always thank a caller for waiting.

CHAPTER 8
THE ORAL CAVITY

I t is very important for each Dental Auxiliary staff member to know all the basic aspects about the procedures performed by a dentist, to work efficiently in a Dental Office. One needs to be familiar with dental terminology (words used to refer to the different parts of the face, mouth, and teeth) because a dentist will use these terms regularly. All this knowledge not only increases the communication ease but also makes the staff member more comfortable in understanding about how the parts and organs that make up the facial structure look and work.

The anatomy of the oral cavity is quite complex, as it consists of several parts. The functions and a description of each of these parts will be explored in this chapter. You'll see how each part of the oral cavity has developed and how each function.

THE PALATE
The palate is often described as the "roof of the mouth." This area makes up the *superior* (upper) portion of the oral cavity as well as the *inferior* (lower) portion of the nasal cavity. The palate itself is a long structure that is covered by several soft tissue components. The palate is divided into two major sections—the hard palate and the soft palate.

The Hard Palate
The hard palate (the bony portion of the mouth's roof) is located in the *anterior* (front) portion of the mouth. A thin epithelial tissue, known as the oral mucosa, covers it. The oral mucosa is made of a dense, highly proliferating tissue that allows it to regenerate quickly.

There is an area in the anterior section of the hard palate that is known as the *palatine rugae*. It is in the area where the mucosa folds into irregular ridges just behind the maxillary (upper) anterior teeth that the palatine rugae can be located. At the end of the palate is a common area that is utilized for both respiration and digestion. This area aids in both the passage of air for respiration and the swallowing of nourishment for digestion. This section is typically the beginning of the throat and is termed the *pharynx.*

Mouth (Oral Cavity)

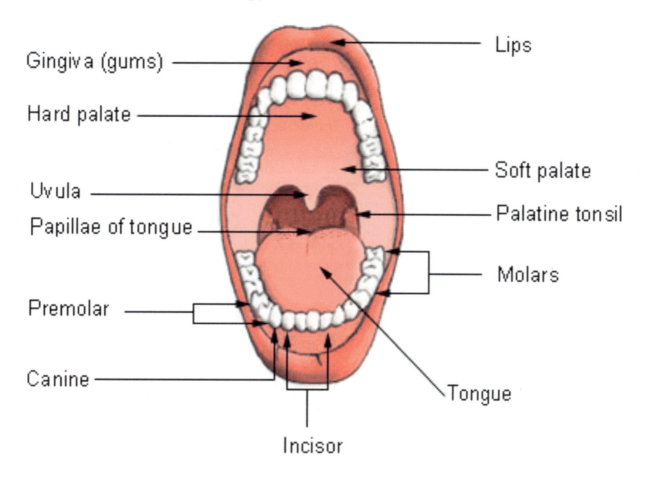

The Soft Palate

The soft palate is located posterior to the hard palate. It is made of soft tissue, including muscle and oral mucosa. The function of the soft palate is to aid in the process of swallowing. The soft palate moves up and back to cover the *nasopharynx* (the portion located behind the nose, above the soft palate) when the swallowing mechanism is initiated. This motion prevents food items from entering the airway, thus preventing choking or aspirating (the breathing in of food particles). The soft palate consists of two main parts—the uvula and the tonsils. The *uvula* is located at the edge of the soft palate, at the center of the entrance of the throat. It consists mainly of lymphatic tissue and assists the body in fighting systemic infections. The *tonsils* are located near the soft palate on both sides of the oropharnyx. The *oropharnyx* extends from the soft palate to the *epiglottis,* which keeps food from entering the *larynx* (the voice box). The oropharynx is the part of the throat that you can see when you look into the mouth. The tonsils are also composed of lymphatic tissue and assist in fighting infections in the body.

The Gag Reflex

The gag reflex is produced in the oral cavity and is basically a protective action of the body. The action itself is produced within the soft palate, the oropharnyx, and the posterior portion of the tongue. This region is covered by a very sensitive mucosa. Any time a foreign body enters this area, the body reacts by closing the posterior oral cavity in order to expel the object from the oral cavity. This action has been termed the gag reflex and is unique in the fact that it is completely involuntary and cannot be controlled.

SALIVARY GLANDS AND DUCTS

The salivary glands are located in the soft tissue surrounding the oral cavity. Their function is to secrete saliva, which is the first step in the process of digestion. Saliva is composed of various proteins manufactured by the salivary glands. Once saliva is made, it has three functions. It aids in digestion through enzymatic breakdown of food; it facilitates swallowing; and it cleanses food debris away from teeth and soft tissue structures.

The salivary glands are divided into four functioning areas—the parotid, the submandibular, the sublingual, and minor salivary glands.

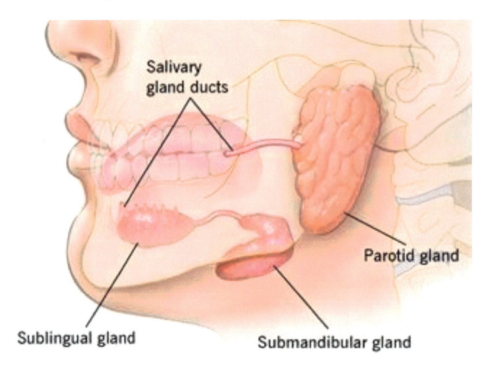

The Parotid Glands

The parotid glands are the largest of the salivary glands. The glands are located on both sides of the oral cavity, just in front of and below each ear. They extend to the lower angle of the mandible (lower jaw area) and are contained within the soft tissues of the cheek. The saliva manufactured by this gland is serous in consistency. It's liquid by nature and is mainly utilized for digestive purposes. The saliva is secreted through a tubule called *Stensen's duct.* This duct opens into the mouth from the cheek just opposite the maxillary (upper jaw area) second molar.

The Submandibular Glands

The submandibular glands are located below the posterior portion of the mandible. The saliva manufactured by these glands is very mucoserous in nature. They are termed the "mixed glands" because their saliva is a cross between a sticky mucous substance and a thin serous consistency. It is utilized for lubrication as well as digestion. These glands secrete saliva through a duct located in the lingual posterior area of the tongue.

The Sublingual Glands

The sublingual glands are the smallest of the three major salivary glands. They are located in the lower anterior floor of the mouth, one on either side of the tongue. The secretions of these glands are mucous like in nature. The function of the secretion is mainly to aid in digestion. The ducts for secretion from these glands are located in the floor of the mouth, under the tongue.

Minor Salivary Glands

Minor salivary glands are located throughout the oral cavity. They may be found on the buccal mucosa, palate, or lips. The secretion from these glands is of a mixed consistency. They secrete directly into the oral cavity without the use of any ducts. They are known as ductless glands.

THE TONGUE

The tongue, which is located on the floor of the oral cavity, is a very specialized set of muscles. It has many functions: it is involved in the action of speech, breathing, and mastication. It is very resilient and flexible in nature, as it consists of both a *dorsal* (top) portion called the *dorsum,* and a *ventral* (bottom) portion.

The Dorsal Surface

The dorsal surface (dorsum) of the tongue is covered with a thick, epithelial tissue covering. The taste buds can be found in the dorsal epithelium. It is interesting to note that there are separate taste buds for different food flavors. For example, there are different taste buds for sweet, salty, and sour flavors. The dorsum of the tongue also contains many valleys and ridges as a normal part of its anatomy.

The Ventral Surface

The ventral surface of the tongue is the underside of the tongue. This is where the tongue attaches to the floor of the mouth. The ventral portion of the tongue is covered by a very delicate and highly vascular epithelium. All the nerve and blood vessels that supply the tongue are within the ventral aspect.

THE FRENUM
The *frenum* is a loose, fibrous connective tissue that is covered by oral mucosa. There are frena located on both the maxillary and mandible arches.

The Maxillary Labial Frenum
The maxillary labial frenum is located between the two front teeth known as the central incisors. The beginning of the frenum starts at the gingiva (gum tissue), passes through the oral mucosa, and ends on the inside (lingual) surface of the lip. The frenum gains significance only if it is attached too closely to the central incisors. In such a situation, it can cause a space between these two teeth, known as a *diastema.* The space can be closed through orthodontic work. However, before this can be accomplished with the use of braces, the frenum may be removed from this area. The frenum may cause the space to reopen if it is not treated correctly.

The Mandibular Labial Frenum
The mandibular labial frenum is located in the lower dental arch, between the two lower central incisors. It is composed of connective tissues. Like the maxillary labial frenum, it can cause a space between the two lower central incisors. Surgical removal is often required in such a situation. However, this procedure is performed less frequently than the maxillary labial frenum procedure. This frenum also begins its attachment in the gingiva and passes through the oral mucosa in order to insert itself into the inner surface of the lower lip.

The Mandibular Lingual Frenum
The mandibular lingual frenum is located underneath the tongue. It originates in the floor of the mouth and passes to the under surface of the mucosa. An abnormality of this frenum can cause a condition known as "tongue-tie." This problem is caused when the frenum attachment limits movement of the tongue. It can be caused either by the frenum being too short or by the frenum being attached to the far anterior of the tongue. Either situation can cause a problem with both speech and swallowing functions. Correction of this problem can be achieved surgically by cutting the frenum in order to allow for free movement of the tongue.

The Buccal Frenum
The buccal frenum can be found on both the maxillary and mandibular arches. These are located in the area of the first premolars on both arches, passing from the gingiva to the inner surface of the cheek. It is very rare that the buccal frenum causes any oral problems or

abnormalities.

The Tissues of the Oral Cavity

The Alveolar Ridge

The alveolar ridge, which supports the teeth in the jaw, can be found in both the maxillary and mandibular arches. It's the bony portion of the upper and lower jaw that houses the tooth sockets. This portion of bone is moderately dense and sponge-like in appearance. A denser bone, known as the cortical plate, supports it. This plate has openings for the passage of vessels and nerves. This area makes up the body of the mandible. Since it is denser on the mandibles, it affects the injection of anesthesia.

A dense bone called the *lamina dura*, a section of the alveolar ridge, lines the tooth socket. The *periodontal ligament,* soft tissue that surrounds the tooth's root and connects it with the bone of the socket wall of the tooth, is attached to the lamina dura.

The Periodontal Ligament

As already mentioned, the periodontal ligament is the soft tissue lining of the tooth socket. Its attachment runs from the lamina dura to the cementum of the tooth. Coarse bundles of fibrous tissue are embedded in the cementum, whose ends are termed *Sharpey's fibers.*

The periodontal ligament has three basic characteristics:

(A) It has specialized cells, which form the cementum, bone, and fibrous tissue specially adopted to support the tooth.

(B) It contains sensory fibers, which are stimulated upon percussion (striking or hitting force) and pressure.

(C) It helps hold the tooth firmly in the tooth socket.

There are five fiber groups of the periodontal ligament, each with its own location and function:

(1) The *alveolar crest fibers* are located at the height of the alveolar bone. Their function is to keep the teeth in their sockets and fight lateral forces.

(2) The *horizontal fibers* are located in the middle third of the tooth and run at right angles to the long axis of the tooth. Their primary purpose is to fight lateral tooth movement.

(3) The *oblique fibers* are at an upward angle towards the coronal part of the tooth. They are located in the apical third (the anatomical area at the end) of the root. Their primary function is to resist *axial* forces (running lengthwise) of the tooth. These fibers are the most numerous and make up the bulk of all fibers.

(4) The *apical fibers* can be found irregularly around the *apex* (end of the tooth root) of the tooth. Their purpose is the resistance of twisting forces. They also protect the blood and nerve supplies of the tooth.

(5) The *interradicular fibers* are located between the roots of teeth. They aid in the axial resistance as well as resistance to tipping.

THE GINGIVA

The gingiva (gum tissue) is the pink-colored tissue that surrounds the teeth and covers the alveolar mucosa. There are two types of gingiva—the *free gingiva* and the *attached gingiva.* The attached gingiva basically covers the alveolar mucosa. It is epithelial on the outside with connective tissue underneath. This gingiva is firmly attached to the underlying alveolar bone.

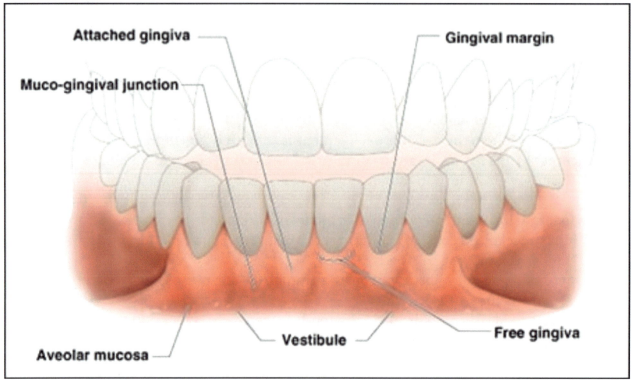

The free gingiva is composed of an epithelial surface with a connective tissue base. It surrounds the tooth buccally, lingually, and interproximally (between adjacent teeth). This tissue extends from the attached gingiva to the area where it attaches to the tooth. This attachment, known as the *epithelial attachment,* is located at the base of the gingival sulcus. The *gingival sulcus* can be found next to the tooth and is formed by free gingival tissue. It is actually the area between the free gingiva and the tooth.

The depth of a healthy gingiva usually does not exceed two millimeters (mm). This area is measured to determine gingival health. A deeper sulcus may indicate gingival inflammation and possibly *periodontal disease* (a general term for the many disorders of the gums). The free gingiva is a coral pink color while the attached gingiva is slightly redder. The difference is due to the fact that there is more vascularization in the attached gingiva. There is an area above the gingiva sulcus that is called the *supragingival area.* This area includes all the structures of the oral cavity. The supragingival area is that area above the free gingiva and not in the gingival sulcus. The *subgingival* is that area below the free gingiva and within the gingival sulcus.

CHAPTER 9
FUNCTIONS OF TEETH

Humans use teeth to tear, grind, and chew food in the first step of digestion. Teeth also play a role in human speech. Additionally, teeth provide structural support to muscles in the face and form the human smile and other facial expressions. So, broadly the main functions of the teeth can be summarized as follows:

1. Helps in mastication.
2. Aids in articulation and speech.
3. Gives shape and beauty to the face.
4. Helps in giving Facial expressions.
5. Like in animals, it may be used for self-protection and attack.

MASTICATORY FUNCTIONS:

One of the main functions of the teeth is the mastication of the food. For the proper and faster digestion of the food, the act of swallowing of the food is preceded by its cutting, chopping, and grinding by the teeth. So, the first step of digestion involves the mouth and teeth. Food enters the mouth and is immediately broken down into smaller pieces by our teeth. Each type of tooth serves a different function in the chewing process. Incisors cut foods when you bite into them. The sharper and longer canines tear food. The premolars, which are flatter than the canines, grind, and mash food. Molars, with their points and grooves, are responsible for the most vigorous chewing. All the while, the tongue helps to push the food up against our teeth. As we chew, salivary glands in the walls and floor of the mouth secrete saliva, which moistens the food and helps break it down even more. Saliva makes it easier to chew and swallow foods (especially dry foods), and it contains enzymes that aid in the digestion of carbohydrates.

Once food has been converted into a soft, moist mass, it is pushed into the throat (or pharynx) at the back of the mouth and is swallowed. When we swallow, the soft palate closes off the nasal passages from the throat to prevent food from entering the nose. So, the process of chewing in the oral cavity not only help in tearing the food into swallowable pieces, but also allow the enzymes and lubricants to be released in the mouth to further digest, or break down, food. Without our teeth - which structurally so strong that they are found to be in great condition in fossils, when the body's skin and bones have disappeared -

we would have to eat nothing but soft, mashed food.

ARTICULATION AND SPEECH:

The mouth - especially the teeth, lips, and tongue - is essential for speech. The teeth, lips, and tongue are used to form words by controlling airflow through the mouth. The tongue, which allows us to taste, also enables us to form words when we speak. The lips that line the outside of the mouth both help hold food in, while we chew, and pronounce words when we talk.

With the lips and tongue, teeth help form words by controlling air flow out of the mouth. The tongue strikes the teeth as certain sounds are made. The *th* sound, for example, is produced by the tongue being placed against the upper row of teeth. If your tongue touches your teeth when you say words with the *s* sound, you may have a slip.

Speech has, during the last 500,000 years, superseded chewing, as main function of the mouth. Simpson (1968) states that "Language has become far more than a means of communication in man. It is also one of the principal means of thought, memory, introspection, problem solving and other mental activities." Recently a very experienced dentist who was watching small children shift the tongue to its natural nose breathing position by singing said "We have to come to accept that the mandible is undergoing a change in function. It is no longer designed for chewing, but for speech".

Human tongues, along with their associated nerves, the respiratory system, and the teeth and lips, are much more versatile than those of other animals, allowing humans the ability to speak unlike any other species on Earth.

FACIAL SHAPE AND BEAUTY:

The importance of the face in social interaction and social intelligence is widely recognized. The teeth play an important role in giving facial fullness and aesthetically pleasant facial shapes. Absence of teeth, due to any reason, not only hampers the masticatory activity of the individual, but also affect the facial features to great extent, affecting the concerned person physiologically, emotionally, and socially.

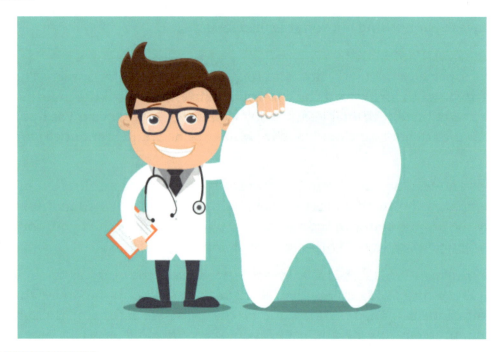

FACIAL EXPRESSIONS:

Your smile, formed by your mouth at your brain's command, is often the first thing people notice when they look at you. It's the facial expression that most engages others. With the help of the teeth - which provide structural support for the face muscles - your mouth also forms your frown and lots of other expressions that show on your face.

Facial expressions can set the mood in many situations and usually tell us what people are thinking or feeling. For example, if we walk toward someone with a smile on our face, we are much more inviting than if we wear an expression of a scowl and pursed lips. Without a mouth and its structures, we would not be able to display our emotions through our expressions.

Our lips, teeth, jaws, cheeks, and facial muscles all play an important role in creating facial expressions. We can make facial expressions because of the complex muscular structure of the face. We have 22 muscles on either side of the face; humans have more facial muscles than any other animal.

SELF PROTECTION AND ATTACK:

This function of teeth is not of much importance in the modern era; however, it has played a significant role in survival of early man and also in the case of animals. Many *carnivorous* (meat-eating) animals, such as tigers, have developed long, sharp teeth for clamping down on and killing prey. Beavers have chisel-like front teeth that they use to cut down large trees for building dams.

CHAPTER 10
PARTS OF THE TEETH

It is very important for every person associated with the work of Dental office to be familiar with the physiology of a tooth as well as the function of each part of the tooth. Three main parts make up a tooth—the crown, the cervix, and the root.

THE CROWN

The crown is the portion of the tooth that is utilized for mastication and is visible in the oral cavity. The dental crown can be divided into two portions—the anatomical crown and the clinical crown.

The *anatomical crown* is the part of the tooth that extends from the incisal or coronal surface to the cervical neck (the cementoenamel junction). It is the part entirely covered by enamel. The *cementoenamel junction* is formed by the line where the enamel of the crown and cementum of the root meet. Another name for this is the *cervical line.*

The *clinical crown* is the section of the tooth from the incisal edge to the crest of the gingival height. The clinical crown is the part you see above the gum line. The clinical crown height can be greater than the anatomical crown height because of periodontal disease, or it can vary with age. Gingival recession can cause exposure of the root, adding length to the clinical crown.

THE CERVIX

The cervix, or neck, is the section of the tooth where the anatomic crown meets the anatomic root. This part of the tooth is also referred to as the cementoenamel junction.

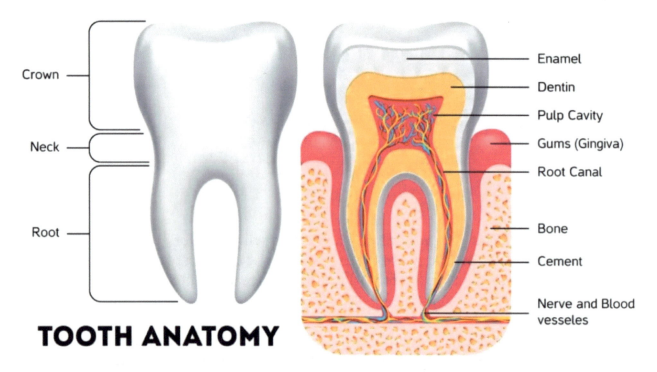

TOOTH ANATOMY

THE ROOT

The root of the tooth is the part that supports the crown and is usually below the gingiva. This section of the tooth is contained within the bony structures of the supporting maxilla and mandible. The root can be divided into two categories—the anatomic root and the clinical root.

The *anatomic root* is the area from the cervix to the apex (the end of the root) of the tooth. It is covered with cementum.

The *clinical root* is the distance from the crestal height of the alveolar bone to the apex of the tooth.

THE APEX

The apex of a tooth is located at the tip of the root. At the end of the root is a small opening —the *apical foramen.* The function of this tiny opening is to "feed" the tooth. The opening allows blood vessels to carry nourishment to a tooth. A second function of the apical foramen is to allow the entrance of nerves to the tooth. This process is known as *innervation* of the tooth.

COMPOSITION OF THE TEETH

A tooth consists of three hard tissue, the enamel, dentin, and cementum, surrounding a soft tissue- the pulp. The pulp is surrounded by dentin on all sides except at the apical foramen, where it is continuous with the periodontal soft tissue.

Enamel

Enamel is the hardest tissue of the entire human body. It is a calcified matrix (material in which something is enclosed), which covers the entire anatomical crown of the tooth and protects the dentin (the inner portion of the tooth). It is formed by epithelial cells. It is made up of 96 percent inorganic (calcium and phosphorous) and four percent organic (carbon compounds) material. Another purpose of enamel is to protect the portion of the tooth, which is exposed to the oral cavity during mastication. When enamel is mature, no further growth or repair takes place.

Cementum

Cementum is a very dense tissue that covers the clinical root of a tooth. It is composed of approximately 55 percent inorganic material (mainly calcium salts) and 45 percent organic material (mainly collagen). Cementum is of light-yellow color and regenerates by forming new layers over older ones. The cementum covers the clinical root and meets the clinical crown at the cementoenamel junction. Sometimes, the cementum and enamel do not meet in a perfect juncture, forming a space which can be sensitive to external stimuli such as heat, cold, chemicals, sweetness, or mechanical stimuli.

The primary function of cementum is to anchor a tooth to the bony wall of the socket. Cementum is formed throughout the life of a tooth. When a fracture of the tooth root takes place, the new cementum formed may replace the lost tissue, helping to repair it. Two types of cementum are usually recognized—primary and secondary.

Dentin

Dentin is the material that makes up the hard structure of a tooth. Dentin is harder than bone but softer than enamel. It is covered by the cementum in the root area and enamel in the crown area. The majority of dentin is composed of inorganic materials (70 percent), mainly calcium. The remaining 30 percent is organic material. Dentin is continually formed throughout the life of the tooth. It forms from the outside of a tooth near the enamel and grows inwards towards the pulp. One of the main functions of dentin is pupal protection. If, for example, the dentin is irritated by bacterial decay, cavity preparation, or wearing away, it changes formation and try to do the repair work by formation of Secondary or Reparative Dentin. The dentin thus formed develops in layer called the *irregular secondary dentin* next to the pupal wall. This dentin is dense and actually forms a layer of insulation over the pulp. An irregular dentin usually forms when severe trauma, such as a deep fracture, is experienced. Dentin continues to develop throughout the life of the tooth. It continues to thicken during this time and eventually invades the pupal chamber. This growth will cause a decrease in the size of the pupal chamber later in a person's life.

Pulp

The pulp is the lifeline of the tooth. The soft tissue of the pulp is found within the hard structures of a tooth. The area that houses the pulp in the coronal (crown) section is called the *pulp chamber.* The area in the root of a tooth that houses the pulp is called the root canal. Finally, the section at the root apex where the pulpal material enters a tooth is called the *apical foramen.* The pulp is composed mainly of loose connective tissue, blood vessels, and nerve materials.

Its function can be divided into the following four categories:
(A) Formation—The external portion of the pulp chamber is lined by odontoblasts (dentin-forming cells). The function of these odontoblasts is in the formation of dentin. The chief function of pulp is to make dentin. The odontoblasts appear as a layer of cells between the pulp and the dentin and are actually part of the pulp.
(B) Nutrition—The pulp supplies the tooth with nutrients necessary for the organic portion of the tooth. It also supplies moisture for the tooth to prevent its desiccation (drying).
(C) Sensation—The pulp has a very extensive nerve supply. Whenever an external stimulus traumatizes a tooth, the pain is transmitted by the nerves and alerts the brain to the presence of a toothache.
(D) Defense—One of the main functions of the pulp is in the formation of secondary dentin for protection whenever an external stimulus causes a pupal reaction. Along with this, the blood supply will form defense cells such as macrophages and fibrocytes for the protection of the tooth.

CHAPTER 11
TOOTH MORPHOLOGY

THE DENTAL ARCHES

The teeth are arranged in two dental arches and these two separate arches, the maxillary, and the mandibular arches, align the human dentition. There are an equal number of teeth in the upper and lower arches. The arrangement of the teeth is symmetrical in the right and the left halves in each arch. The teeth of one half of the jaw are exact mirror image of the other half. Thus, in each arch there are 10 deciduous teeth and 16 permanent teeth. In other words, each of four quadrants of the jaw will have 5 deciduous and 8 permanent teeth.

The maxillary arch is located in the upper portion of the oral cavity. The permanent dentition contains 16 teeth in each arch, including two each of central, laterals, canines or cuspids, first and second premolars, and first, second, and third molars. The maxillary arch is firmly attached to the base of the skull. The mandibular arch is located in the mandible or lower jaw.

In the mandibular arch, the permanent dentition contains 16 teeth of the same variety as those found in the maxillary arch. The mandibular arch is movable through the lower jaw. The closing of the jaw causes the two arches to meet, allowing the chewing process to occur. The arches can be further divided into *quadrants*. Each arch contains two quadrants, a right and a left. The median line forms these quadrants. This line is a bisection starting between the central incisors and continuing straight back towards the posterior oral cavity, ending at the beginning of the oropharynx. Each quadrant contains eight teeth—one central incisor, one lateral incisor, one canine or cuspid, two premolars, and three molars. There is a specific pattern formed as the jaw opens and closes called *occlusion*. This pattern is formed when the maxillary and mandibular arches meet. Occlusion is made possible only by the ability of the lower jaw to move. The hinge, which makes such movement possible, is termed the *temporomandibular joint.*

TEMPROMANDIBULAR JOINT (TMJ)

The temporomandibular joint, abbreviated TMJ, is the movable hinge where the maxilla and mandible meet. The TMJ receives its name from the two bases that meet at this area, the temporal base and the mandible. The joint itself consists of three major bony parts. The *articular eminence* is the raised section of the temporal bone that guides the mandible. The *glenoid fossa* is an oval depression of the temporal base that houses the condyloid process. The *condyloid process* is the head of the mandible that fits into the glenoid fossa. The condyloid process articulates with the fossa in the temporal bones to form the temporomandibular joint. The TMJ has connective tissue and muscle incorporated into its working mechanism. The muscles of mastication assist in holding the TMJ in place. They also help in the functioning of the joint. The *meniscus* (also known as the articular disc) consists of tough connective tissue. The disc aids the condyle in sliding along the articular eminence. It fits into the glenoid fossa when the jaw is closed. The capsular ligament is dense, fibrous connective tissue, which totally encloses the TMJ. It attaches to the neck of the condyle and the temporal bone. Its functions are in support and protection from trauma. The movement that occurs when the lower jaw opens causes the condyle to rotate within the glenoid fossa. This movement, called *rotational movement,* occurs when the jaw opens to approximately two-thirds of its capacity. As the mandible continues to open, it enters the transitional movement of the TMJ. During transitional movement, the condyle slides down the articular eminence on the articular disc. This process causes the jaw to move down and forward to create a wider opening. A condition known as *TMJ syndrome* occurs when there is an abnormality within the joint. This condition can include degeneration of the articular disc, eminence, or condyle. More often, it's a result of a combination of several problems. The most severe TMJ problems must be treated surgically.

TOOTH SURFACES
There are several characteristics of the external appearance of a tooth. The following section describes the tooth surfaces of both the anterior and posterior teeth.

Proximal
The proximal surface or contact is formed by the contact of two adjacent teeth. The mesial surface of one tooth contacts the distal surface of the adjacent tooth to form the proximal contact. The two surfaces that come into contact with each other are called the proximal surfaces.

The *mesial surface* is the side of the tooth closest to the middle (midline) of the dental arch. The *distal surface* is the side of the tooth that is farthest away from the arch middle (midline).

Interproximal Area
The interproximal area is formed by the proximal contact of adjacent teeth. The area above the proximal contact, towards the gingiva, is the interproximal space. This space is usually filled with unattached gingiva.

Lingual Surface
The lingual surface is the area of the tooth, both anterior and posterior, that is closest to the tongue.

Labial Surface
The labial surface is the portion of the anterior tooth that faces the lip.

Buccal Surface
The buccal surface of the tooth is the portion of the posterior tooth that faces the cheek.

Facial Surface
The facial surface is a generic term for both the posterior and anterior teeth. The facial surface refers to both the buccal and labial surfaces of the teeth collectively.

Occlusal Surface
The surface of the tooth that occludes with the tooth of the opposite arch is known as occlusal surface. In other words, the occlusal surface is the section of the posterior teeth that's utilized as the actual biting and chewing surface.

Incisal Edge
The incisal edge is the portion of the anterior teeth used for tearing or incision of the food items. It is the very edge of the anterior teeth.

Vestibular Surface
Vestibular is a collective term which refers to the facial surface of an anterior or posterior tooth. Therefore, vestibular identifies either a labial or a buccal surface and is interchangeable when coding for insurance or in written documentation.

Each tooth surface is identified by the *first letter of the name of the surface*. For example: **MODBL** identifies the surfaces: mesial, occlusal, distal, buccal, and lingual. The suffix **al** of each word identifies the term as an adjective and describes the relationship of the surface to the dental arch.

TYPES OF TEETH
Human dentition consists of two sets of teeth: (1) Primary, Deciduous or Milk dentition, and (2) Permanent, Secondary or Succedaneous dentition.

Based on form and function, the teeth may be divided into three classes in case of primary dentition (Incisors, Canines and Molars) and four classes in case of permanent dentition

(Incisors, Canines, Premolars and Molars).

STAGES OF DENTITION

The dentition can be roughly divided into three periods and stages:

(1) **Stage of Primary Dentition:** During this period only the deciduous teeth are present in the oral cavity. This stage starts at about 6 months of age with the eruption of first primary teeth in the mouth, and last till the age of 6 years, when permanent teeth starts erupting.

(2) **Stage of Mixed Dentition:** This stage generally last from 6 years to 13 years of age. During this stage both the deciduous and the permanent teeth are present in the oral cavity.

(3) **Stage of permanent Dentition:** This stage lasts from 13 years of age till the individual losses all of his permanent teeth. During this stage only permanent teeth are present in the oral cavity.

PRIMARY DENTITION

The primary teeth are the first set of teeth that develop in the human oral cavity. They're often referred to as the baby teeth or the deciduous teeth. There are 20 primary teeth —10 maxillary and 10 mandibular. They perform several important functions, including aiding in the chewing and digestion of food, and aiding in speech and pronunciation. The primary dentition guides the eruption of the permanent teeth. One of the most important factors in the eruption of the permanent teeth is that the proper space required is available. This space is maintained by the retention and timely exfoliation (shedding) of the primary dentition. So, the primary teeth also function as the Natural Space Maintainer for the permanent dentition. Any premature or delayed exfoliation of the primary dentition may cause problems with secondary tooth eruption.

Teeth of the Maxillary Arch

Primary Central Incisor

The primary central incisor is located in the front of the maxillary arch. It is utilized for cutting and dividing food items. Eventually, it is replaced with the permanent central incisors.

Primary Lateral Incisor

The primary lateral incisor performs the same function as the central incisor. However, it's slightly smaller than the central incisor. The permanent lateral incisor replaces it.

Primary Cuspid (also known as Canine)

The primary cuspid (primary canine) is the cornerstone of the primary dentition. It is utilized for tearing and shredding of food particles. It also maintains the arch integrity. Premature loss of this tooth can cause arch disharmony. The primary cuspid (canine) is replaced by the permanent cuspid (canine). The cuspids, along with the central and lateral incisors, are called the anterior teeth.

Primary First Molar
The primary first molar is used for grinding and pulverizing food. It resembles the permanent first molar. However, it is replaced by the permanent first premolar.

Primary Second Molar
The primary second molar is the largest of the primary teeth. It helps to grind food. The permanent second premolar eventually replaces this tooth.

Teeth of the Mandibular Arch

Primary Mandibular Central Incisor
The primary mandibular central incisor is the smallest tooth in the primary dentition. The mandibular permanent central incisor replaces it, which is also the smallest in the mandibular permanent arch.

Primary Mandibular Lateral Incisor
The primary mandibular lateral incisor resembles the central incisor. However, it is slightly larger than central incisor. The permanent lateral incisor replaces this tooth.

Primary Mandibular Cuspid (also known as Canine)
The primary mandibular cuspid (canine) serves the same function as the maxillary canine, that of tearing and shredding food. It causes stabilization of the mandibular arch. It is replaced by the permanent cuspid.

Primary Mandibular First Molar
The primary mandibular first molar grinds and breaks up food items. It is eventually replaced by the permanent first premolar.

Primary Mandibular Second Molar
The primary mandibular second molar is the largest mandibular tooth. The permanent second premolar eventually takes the place of this tooth.

THE ERUPTION OF PRIMARY DENTITION

Tooth Eruption Age (in months)

Maxillary Arch (Upper teeth)
Central Incisor 8–12 months
Lateral Incisor 9–13 months
Cuspid 16–22 months
First Molar 13–19 months
Second Molar 25–33 months

Mandibular Arch (Lower teeth)
Central Incisor 6–10 months
Lateral Incisor 10–16 months
Cuspid 17–23 months
First Molar 14–18 months
Second Molar 23–31 months

THE MIXED DENTITION

The mixed dentition refers to the presence of primary and permanent teeth together in the oral cavity. This usually occurs between the ages of five and thirteen years as primary teeth are exfoliated, and permanent teeth erupt. It is during the time of mixed dentition that dental abnormalities become apparent. Dental conditions such as missing permanent teeth or malformed teeth become visible. It is at this time that skeletal and dental malformations will come into view. An orthodontist should be consulted as soon as any occlusal disharmonies are discovered.

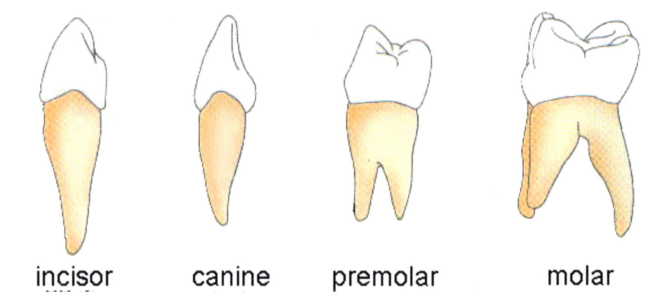

incisor   canine   premolar   molar

THE PERMANENT DENTITION

The permanent dentition consists of the permanent teeth in the human oral cavity, those teeth which remain throughout one's adult life. The permanent dentition is also known as the secondary dentition. The permanent dentition numbers 32 teeth altogether. There are 16 teeth in both the maxillary and mandibular arches. Each arch can be further divided into anterior and posterior teeth. The anterior teeth are the front six teeth, including two lateral incisors, two central incisors, and two cuspids. There are 10 posterior teeth in each arch, including four premolars and six molars. There are very specific functions of both the anterior and posterior teeth. Teeth generally erupt during a time-period (age range) for that particular tooth.

Maxillary Central Incisor
The maxillary central incisors are the two most anterior teeth in the maxillary arch. The median line bisects them. They are also the first teeth to be found in each of the maxillary quadrants. This tooth has a sharp incisal edge for cutting food. This edge has developmental mamelons upon eruption. Mamelons are prominences at the incisal edge of a newly erupted tooth. These mamelons wear away with the use of the tooth. This tooth is the widest of all the anterior teeth.

Maxillary Lateral Incisor
The lateral incisors are the next teeth to be found in the maxillary arch. They are adjacent to the central incisors and have the same form and function. They have a cutting edge and are utilized primarily for ripping and shredding food items. Interestingly, they are the smallest and weakest of the teeth in the maxillary arch.

Maxillary Cuspid/Canine
The cuspid (canine) is the longest and strongest rooted tooth in the maxillary arch. It's often referred to as the "eye tooth." The purpose of this tooth is to aid in ripping and tearing food. It is a very strong tooth and forms the cornerstone of the arch. The shape and function of the cuspid (canine) starts the transition into the posterior portion of the arch. The cuspid (canine) is the last anterior tooth and is located just distal to both maxillary lateral incisors. The root is single and is the longest root in the arch.

Maxillary First Premolar
The maxillary first premolar (or first bicuspid) is considered the first posterior tooth. It is double-rooted and double-cusped. It is utilized for the grinding of food on its occlusal surface. It is located distal to the cuspid on both sides of the arch. This tooth is called a premolar because it is in front of the molars.

Maxillary Second Premolar
The maxillary second premolar is a single-rooted tooth. It has two cusps that are basically of the same size. It has a slightly rounded, molar-like occlusal surface. The occlusal surface is the horizontal surface of the posterior teeth. Its function is in grinding and tearing food. The second premolar continues the transition to a wider occlusal table in the molar area. It can be located just distal to the first premolars on both sides of the arch.

Maxillary First Molar
The maxillary first molar is the largest tooth in the oral cavity. It has three roots—two buccal and one lingual or palatal. It also has four cusps—two buccal and two lingual. It may also contain an accessory cusp that would be located lingually. This cusp is termed the Cusp of Carabelli and may vary in size and shape. The maxillary first molar is sometimes called the six-year molar due to the time of its initial eruption. It is located distal to the second

premolar. The function of the maxillary first molar is in fine grinding of food for deglutition (swallowing).

Maxillary Second Molar

The maxillary second molar closely resembles the maxillary first molar. However, this molar is smaller in diameter and the Cusp of Carabelli is not present. The function of this tooth is the same as the maxillary first molar—namely, fine grinding of food. It is sometimes called the twelve-year molar due to its eruption time. The maxillary second molar is located just distal to the maxillary first molar. It is the seventh tooth from the midline and, therefore, the seventh tooth in each maxillary quadrant.

Maxillary Third Molar

The maxillary third molar is the eighth and last tooth in the maxillary arch. It can vary in shape and size dramatically. It can have a single fused root or many roots. Its occlusal surface is generally heart-shaped, but this can greatly differ. It is also known as the wisdom tooth due to the fact that its eruption time occurs in later years, usually when a person is 16 to 22 years old.

Mandibular Central Incisor

The mandibular central incisor is located on both sides of the median line. It is the smallest tooth in the oral cavity. It also has the most symmetrical design. It has no mamelons or developmental grooves. This tooth is the first tooth of both quadrants of the mandibular arch.

Mandibular Lateral Incisor

The mandibular lateral incisor closely resembles the central incisor. It's shaped similarly. However, it is larger in all dimensions. It is the second tooth of each mandibular quadrant and just distal to the mandibular central incisor.

Mandibular Cuspid (Canine)

The mandibular cuspid (canine) resembles the maxillary cuspid (canine). However, this tooth has a shorter root and a longer, wider crown. It functions as the lower arch stabilizer. It is the last anterior tooth, located just distal to the lateral incisor. The root is not as long as the maxillary cuspid's (canine's) and is flatter.

Mandibular First Premolar

The mandibular first premolar (also known as bicuspid) is the first tooth of the posterior dentition. Its function is grinding. It has a large functional buccal cusp and a smaller, relatively nonfunctional lingual cusp. It is located distal to the cuspid and is the fourth tooth from the median line.

Mandibular Second Premolar

The mandibular second premolar (sometimes called bicuspid) has three cusps—one larger buccal cusp and two smaller lingual cusps. Its primary purpose is in the grinding of food. It is slightly larger than the first premolar. The second premolar can be found just distal to the first premolar in both quadrants and is the fifth tooth from the median line.

Mandibular First Molar

The mandibular first molar is the largest tooth in the mandibular arch and is the first permanent tooth to erupt. It has two roots—one mesial and one distal. It has five cusps on the occlusal surface. It is just distal to the second premolar.

Mandibular Second Molar

The mandibular second molar is located distal to the first molar. It is similar in function to the first molar. It has four cusps—two buccal and two lingual. The second molar also has two roots—one distal and the other mesial, both smaller than those of the first molar.

Mandibular Third Molar

The mandibular third molar is the last tooth in each mandibular quadrant. It is sometimes called the wisdom tooth, just like its maxillary counterpart. The third molar can have many distinctive shapes, forms, and sizes. It may have four or five cusps like the first and second molars. The roots may either be fused together or widely spread apart. The third molar usually has a mesial angle.

THE ERUPTION OF PERMANENT DENTITION

Tooth Eruption Age (in years)

Maxillary Arch
Central Incisor 7–8 years
Lateral Incisor 7–9 years
Cuspids 11–13 years
First Premolar 9–11 years
Second Premolar 10–12 years
First Molar 6–7 years
Second Molar 11–14 years
Third Molar 16–22 years

Mandibular Arch
Central Incisor 6–8 years
Lateral Incisor 7–8 years
Cuspid 9–10 years
First Premolar 10–12 years
Second Premolar 11–12 years
First Molar 6–7 years
Second Molar 11–14 years
Third Molar 16–22 years

ANATOMIC CHARACTERISTICS SHOWN BY DIFFERENT TEETH TYPES
PERMANENT TEETH

FEATURES COMMON TO ALL INCISORS:
1. They have a single, cone-shaped, tapering root.
2. The incisal edge of newly erupted teeth shows mamelons.
3. The crowns are triangular when viewed from proximal aspect.
4. The crowns do not have any linear faults.
5. The facial surface is convex, and the lingual surface is concave in the incisal half.

FEATURES COMMON TO ALL CANINES:
1. They have a single root, which is longest and strongest of all the teeth.
2. They have a single conical cusp.
3. They have a functional lingual surface.

FEATURES COMMON TO ALL PREMOLAR TEETH:
1. They have two or more cusps.
2. They have one buccal cusp and one or more lingual cusps.

FEATURES COMMON TO ALL MOLAR TEETH:
1. They are the largest teeth of dentition.
2. They have a box like crown with five surfaces. The occlusal surface is adopted for grinding.
3. They have strong and long roots to withstand grinding stress.

DECIDUOUS TEETH

FEATURES COMMON TO ALL INCISORS:
1. They have a single, cone-shaped, tapering root.
2. They are smaller than permanent incisors.
3. The cervical margin in prominent.
4. Mamelons at the incisal margin is not seen.
5. The cingulum is relatively more prominent.

FEATURES COMMON TO ALL CANINES:
1. They resemble permanent canines, though are shorter.
2. Mesial incisal ridge is longer than distal incisal ridge.

FEATURES COMMON TO ALL MOLAR TEETH:
1. They have two to three roots.
2. The roots are divergent.
3. They show a prominent cervical bulge buccally.

4. The occlusal surface is relatively narrow bucco-lingually.
5. Root trunk is absent.
6. Show a constricted cervical region.

ANATOMIC LANDMARKS OF THE TEETH

Teeth can differ from person to person, as well as within the oral cavity. However, all teeth contain some of the same developmental anatomical landmarks. The following section presents some of these common characteristics.

Pits

A pit is a small, deep point on the occlusal or buccal surface of both maxillary and mandibular molars. Pits usually occur where several developmental lines converge. It is usually situated at the junction of developmental grooves or at terminals of these grooves.

Fissures

A fissure is a linear fault along a developmental groove (line). Fissures are formed by the convergence of the separate enamel lobes. Lobes are developmental segments of a tooth. When lobes do not join correctly on the occlusal surface, deep grooves are formed. These grooves are called fissures.

Fossa

The fossa is a rounded depression on the surface of tooth. It occurs commonly on occlusal surfaces of posterior teeth and lingual surfaces of anterior teeth. Occlusal fossae may be either central or triangular.

Developmental Grooves

Groove is a linear depression on the surface of the tooth. Developmental grooves (lines on the surface of the tooth) are the areas formed where the enamel lobes join on the occlusal surface. This union is generally at a smooth and complete joint. Therefore, it differs from a fissure in composition. A developmental groove denotes the endence of coalescence between the primary parts of the crown or root. It may be *Buccal* or *Lingual* and are seen on buccal and lingual surfaces of posterior teeth.

Lobe

The lobe is one of the main morphological divisions of the crown of a tooth. It is one of the primary centers of calcification. Cusps and mamelons are representative of lobes.

Cingulum

The cingulum is a rounded, raised portion of enamel. It is located on the lingual section of anterior teeth. It is usually located in the cervical third of lingual surface of the tooth.

Mamelon

A mamelon is one of the three prominent, rounded protuberances of enamel located on the incisal edge of each newly erupted incisor. As the tooth is utilized, the mamelons wear down to a flat, functional incisal edge.

Cusps

The cusps are raised, pointed, or rounded elevations of enamel. They are found on the occlusal surface of cuspids, premolars, and molars. It has an apex and four ridges.

Inclined Plane

The inclined plane is a sloping area on occlusal surfaces of premolars and molars. Each cusp has two inclined planes.

Ridges

A ridge is long, elevated portion on the surface of a tooth. It is called *Buccal, incisal,* and *marginal ridge* depending on its location. There are four basic ridges found on either molars, premolars, or incisors.

(i) A *marginal ridge* is a raised, rounded border of enamel that forms the mesial and distal margins of posterior teeth. Also, the marginal ridge forms the mesial and distal margins of the lingual surfaces of anterior teeth.

(ii) The *triangular ridge* descends from the cusp tip of bicuspids and molars to the occlusal depressions called fossa. There are not as many triangular ridges on a tooth as there are cusps.

(iii) The *oblique ridge* is a raised portion of enamel. It runs diagonally across the occlusal surface of molars from mesio-lingual to disto-buccal.

(iv) The *transverse ridge* is a raised portion of enamel. The buccal and lingual triangular ridges form it. It is found on both premolars and molars.

Sulcus

The sulcus is a long depression on the surface of a tooth, the inclines of which meet at an angle.

Tubercle

A tubercle is a small, rounded elevation of enamel on the crown of a tooth.

TOOTH IDENTIFICATION AND NUMBERING SYSTEMS

Tooth Identification

Systems of tooth identification have been designed to facilitate ease of diagnosis, recording information on the dental chart and performing treatment. In addition to aiding in diagnosis and treatment, identification systems enhance the efficiency of dental claims adjudication. A DOA can identify where the tooth is located in the mouth, whether it is a primary or permanent tooth, and the type of restoration involved. Information is recorded by the insurance company to prevent the duplication of claim payment.

There are a variety of methods of identification available to the dental professional, and the three most commonly used systems are discussed in this book.

A. International Tooth Numbering System OR FDI World Dental Federation notation
B. Palmer System
C. Universal Tooth Numbering System

International (FDI World Dental Federation notation) and Palmer systems are commonly used in Canada. Universal system is widely used in United States and some countries in Europe.

Numbering Systems

A. International Tooth Numbering System

International Dental Federation (FDI) tooth notation is commonly used in dental practice in many countries. FDI tooth notation is widely used by dentists internationally to associate information to a specific tooth. It is widely used by dentists to associate a specific tooth by two digits. This system is the most efficient and easy to use. It is often called the two-digit numbering system. FDI tooth notation is a two-digit system where one digit shows quadrant in which the tooth is located, and the second one shows the location of the tooth in the quadrant. The first digit also indicates whether the tooth is permanent or primary. This system also provides a means to distinguish between a permanent and a primary tooth.

To understand this system, it is necessary to divide the mouth into four quadrants. An adult dentition consists of 32 teeth; therefore, each quadrant will contain eight teeth. Beginning at the midline of the upper right quadrant, the teeth are as follows:

central incisor
lateral incisor
cuspid
first bicuspid (premolar)
second bicuspid (premolar)
first molar (6-year molar)
second molar (12-year molar)
third molar or wisdom tooth

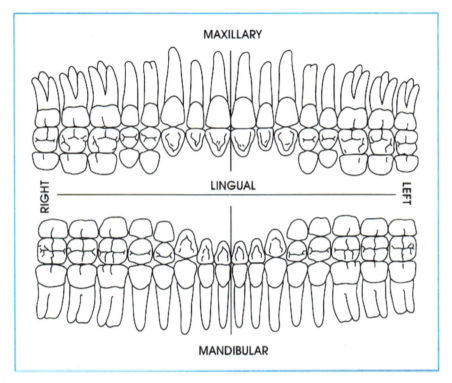

Beginning in the upper right quadrant, this is identified as quadrant # 1. Proceeding in a clockwise direction, the upper left quadrant is identified as # 2. The lower left quadrant is then labeled as quadrant # 3. The lower right quadrant is quadrant # 4.

The second number in the two-digit International Tooth Numbering System identifies location of the tooth in the quadrant. Hence, beginning at the midline, the central incisor is tooth no. 1. The lateral incisor would be tooth no. 2. The cuspid is no. 3. The first bicuspid is no. 4. The second bicuspid is no. 5. The first molar is no. 6, the second molar is no. 7. The third molar is no. 8.

As per this system-
- Upper right central incisor- is identified as tooth no.1.1 (pronounced one-one) according to this tooth numbering system.
- Upper left first bicuspid is tooth no. 2.4 (two-four).
- Lower left lateral incisor- is tooth no. 3.2 (three-two), and
- Lower right first molar- is tooth no. 4.6 (four-six).

Permanent Teeth														
			Upper Right					Upper Left						
18	17	16	15	14	13	12	11	21	22	23	24	25	26	27	28
48	47	46	45	44	43	42	41	31	32	33	34	35	36	37	38
			Lower Right					Lower Left						

Primary teeth									
		Upper Right			Upper Left				
55	54	53	52	51	61	62	63	64	65
85	84	83	82	81	71	72	73	74	75
		Lower Right			Lower Left				

International Tooth Numbering system for Primary Dentition

The International Tooth Numbering System also helps to distinguish between a permanent and a primary tooth. The primary dentition contains only 20 teeth; therefore, there are five teeth in each quadrant. Each quadrant is identified by number beginning in the upper right quadrant and numbering in a clockwise direction.

The main difference, however, is that the upper right quadrant is now quadrant # 5. The upper left quadrant is quadrant # 6, the lower left quadrant is quadrant # 7, and the lower right quadrant is quadrant # 8.

Beginning at the midline, the central incisor is tooth no. 1. The lateral incisor is tooth no. 2, the cuspid is tooth no. 3, and the primary molars are no. 4 and no. 5. *For example*, the upper right primary central incisor is tooth no. 5.1. The upper left primary lateral incisor is tooth no. 6.2. The lower left primary cuspid is tooth no. 7.3. The lower right primary first molar is tooth no. 8.4.

B. Palmer Identification System

The Palmer system presents a more graphic illustration tooth location in each quadrant. This system uses a symbol to indicate the quadrant. It is helpful to think of the vertical line as the midline and the horizontal line as the transverse plane. To identify the left and right teeth the brackets are introduced in it. The brackets are put like this (⌋ ⌊ ⌐ ⌐). The brackrt enclose the tooth number to easily identify the quadrant and the tooth number. Beginning at the midline, in the adult dentition, the teeth are numbered 1 to 8 in each quadrant.

Palmer notation

Permanent Teeth		
upper right	upper left	
8⌋ 7⌋ 6⌋ 5⌋ 4⌋ 3⌋ 2⌋ 1⌋	L¹ L² L³ L⁴ L⁵ L⁶ L⁷ L⁸	
8⌐ 7⌐ 6⌐ 5⌐ 4⌐ 3⌐ 2⌐ 1⌐	Γ₁ Γ₂ Γ₃ Γ₄ Γ₅ Γ₆ Γ₇ Γ₈	
lower right	lower left	
Deciduous teeth (baby teeth)		
upper right	upper left	
E⌋ D⌋ C⌋ B⌋ A⌋	ᴸA ᴸB ᴸC ᴸD ᴸE	
E⌐ D⌐ C⌐ B⌐ A⌐	ΓA ΓB ΓC ΓD ΓE	
lower right	lower left	

Palmer Identification System is an efficient method to identify through graphic representation of the tooth location. For the primary dentition, the Palmer's system uses lower case letters starting from the midline of each quadrant. These letters, along with the quadrant indicators, identify the precise location and type of tooth. To identify the left and right teeth the brackets are introduced in it. The brackets are put like this (⌋ ⌊ ⌐ ⌐)

C. Universal Tooth Numbering System

The Universal Tooth Numbering System is a method of numbering teeth that is widely accepted in the United States and Europe. This system is uncomplicated but is not as easy to use as the FDI System. In this system, as the dentist begins the examination in the upper right quadrant at the location of the third molar, each tooth is numbered from 1 to 32 (in the adult dentition) proceeding in a clockwise direction from that point. For example, maxillary right third molar is tooth no. 1 and, continuing around to the mandibular right side, the third molar is tooth no. 32.

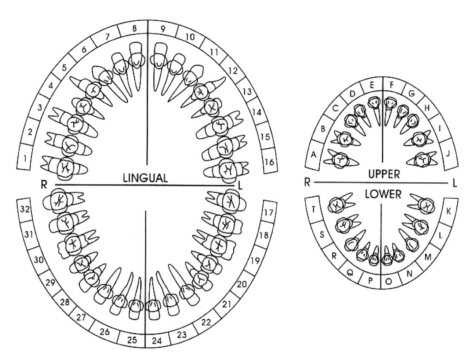

In this system the primary teeth are identified by letters instead of numbers. Beginning at the maxillary right second primary molar and continuing in a clockwise direction, the first tooth is identified with the letter A. The next molar is B, the cuspid is C, the lateral is D, and the incisor is E.

This identification system works well when the quadrants are learnt, and the teeth are counted. However, a problem with this system can occur if a tooth is extracted and the adjacent tooth drifts into that position. This makes identification difficult. Also, when any adult patient does not have all four third molars, this may create problem with identification.

CHAPTER 12
FACTORS AFFECTING THE SELECTION OF DENTAL MATERIALS FOR USE IN ORAL CAVITY

The selection of a proper material for use in oral cavity is very important for the long-term success of the treatment. There are several factors that play an important role in selection of an ideal dental restorative material for the use in a particular patient. However, to understand the various factors, which guide us in the selection of proper material to be used for restoration of the teeth in oral cavity, we should be aware of the objective of the filling or the restoration.

OBJECTS OF FILLING MATERIALS
The various object of the filling material can be broadly outlined as follows:
1. Prevention of recurrence of dental caries (decay)
2. Arrest of loss of tooth structure from caries
3. Establishment of proper occlusion
4. Accomplishment of ideal aesthetics
5. Resistance against masticatory forces
6. Maintenance of normal interproximal spaces and contact point.

To achieve the above-mentioned objects, we need to select the proper dental material, taking into the consideration the various factors, expectations, environment, and forces to which the selected material will be exposed.

FACTORS AFFECTION THE SELECTION OF MATERIAL
Some of the important factors, which directly affect THE selection of the Dental materials for use in the oral cavity, are as follows:

Masticatory Forces
Digestion is the process of breaking down food both mechanically (physically) and chemically. This process begins in mouth, where food is mechanically broken down into small pieces through biting, chewing, and grinding actions. So, any restoration of the tooth is continuously exposed to these heavy masticatory loads in the oral cavity. The oral environment is particularly conducive to breaking down or dissolving materials. The

combination of saliva and the mechanical forces of biting /chewing that begin the digestive process require any dental restorative (repairing) materials to be strong and insoluble. Those biting forces average 28,000 pounds per square inch (psi). Because of this, the amalgam and composites used extensively as restorative material in modern dentistry, feature strengths in excess of 85,000 psi.

Acidity

The oral environment is exposed to different kinds of acids. Enzymes found in saliva, which help in digestion of food chemically, are acidic in nature. There are acids in many of the common foods. Ascorbic acid, for example, is found in citrus fruits. In addition of acidic nature of many food items, the normal bacteria present in the mouth also liberate acids. Because acids accelerate the breakdown of materials, teeth and the restorative materials must be insoluble and resistant to the acidic substances. Many of the early generation of nonmetallic restoratives used to show deterioration over time, dissolving away in this acidic environment.

However, on the contrary, because of the properties of the metals used in dental amalgam, the amalgam restoration corrodes in a "controlled fashion" that could improve the marginal seal of the restoration.

Temperature

Every day the oral cavity is exposed to different temperatures as we eat and drink foods that are so varied in temperature, from hot drinks to ice cream. Teeth expand marginally when exposed to hot food and contract on exposure to clod food. Therefore, any restorative materials placed in a tooth must not only be able to withstand extreme temperature changes, but also closely match the thermal expansion and contraction of the tooth. If the difference in thermal expansion between the tooth and restorative material is too great, the margin between the restorative material and tooth can open, creating a microscopic space, which may lead to microleakage.

Microleakage

Microleakage is the leakage of very small amounts of fluid, debris, and/or microorganisms (e.g., bacteria or viruses) into a microscopic space between a tooth and its restorative material. As just mentioned, differences in thermal expansion between a tooth and restorative material can create such a space. The inability of dental restorative material to seal the margins of a cavity preparation also can result in a microscopic space at the junction. So, improper bonding of restorative material with the tooth surface may also cause microleakage. Continued microleakage will lead to restoration failure, secondary caries(decay) and pulpal irritation causing sensitivity or permanent pulpal damage.

Sensitivity

If microleakage is severe, sensitivity of the tooth (pain in the tooth that lasts a short period of time) and failure of the restoration may occur. Another type of sensitivity may occur when two different metals are present in the mouth. An ionic or galvanic reaction may occur in this moist environment, producing a small electric current. This reaction can cause a galvanic shock and associated sensitivity. This situation particularly happens, when two different types of metals are used for restoration of two opposing teeth. This sensitivity may also occur when a metal eating utensil touches a metallic restoration. Another sensitivity is produced when proper sedative layer is not used below the metallic fillings causing the transmission of hot or cold sensation to the underlying living tissue of the tooth.

Retention
Retention of the restoration must be achieved by mechanical and/or adhesive methods. Traditional restorative techniques rely on mechanical retention. They must take into consideration the factors of biting stress and tooth structure removal. Adhesive retention (bonding) is complicated by the moist environment of the mouth, varying thermal expansions of materials involved, and the difference associated with the inorganic and organic materials of the tooth structure and restorative.

Biocompatibility
The biocompatibility of the restorative material is extremely important. The material must be harmless to the teeth and oral tissues to be suitable. The materials must not be irritating, allergenic, poisonous, or harmful to the body.

Esthetics
It is also one of the important factor or criteria for selection of proper restorative material as generally the main concern of the dental patients are about how they will look after their dentist repairs or replaces their teeth. They want to maintain a pleasing appearance or esthetics. Permanent restorations in the posterior of the mouth are not generally visible in a normal smile, so the silver color of dental amalgam was traditionally accepted. However, restorations in the anterior regions of the mouth demand a tooth shade matching the individuals existing dentition. The modern composite materials offer nearly unlimited color matching and have excellent color stability.

Age of the Patient
Age of the patient is also an important factor taken into consideration, before selecting some material to be used in the particular patient. The material, which may be good for short-term use in deciduous teeth of a small child, may not be the ideal material for use in a permanent tooth of a young patient. The structural difference, particularly of the pulpal tissues and the size of dentinal tubules in deciduous and permanent teeth, also affect the decision of selection of material. Similarly, in a very old patient, who may be having more reparative dentin formation with the ageing, giving more pulpal tissue protection, the material choice may be different.

Cost Factor

The cost or economics of the material also play an important role in selection of restorative material, particularly in case of developing countries with large population under the poverty line. Sometimes, even the material may be an ideal choice on the basis of its physical and chemical properties, due to the cost factor and inability of the patient to afford the cost of the procedure; the material may not be used in that particular patient.

IDEAL REQUIREMENT OF THE FILLING MATERIAL

After taking into consideration the objective of the dental filling (or restoration) and the various factors responsible for selection of the material, we can outline the following requirements of an ideal filling material:

1. Indestructibility in the oral fluids.
2. It should not damage or irritate the pulp or any other underlying tissues.
3. Good adaptability to cavity walls.
4. Harmonious in color.
5. Resistance to masticatory or occluding forces.
6. Resistance to attrition and good edge strength.
7. Non-conductivity to thermal or electric changes.
8. Free from Postoperative dimensional changes.
9. It should be biocompatible.
10. It should have same amount of thermal expansion or contraction as that of natural tooth structure.
11. It should not be very expensive.
12. It should be easy to use for the operator.

CHAPTER 13
DENTAL AMALGAM

One of dentistry's oldest and most widely used restorative material is dental amalgam. Amalgam is without a doubt a restorative material with an excellent clinical record and has served hundreds of millions of patients successfully for more than 100 years. Amalgam's reputation as a relatively inexpensive, forgiving, and durable restorative material is well deserved and well documented.

ADVANTAGES

Though, the use of Silver amalgam has declined considerably in recent time, but still, it is continuing to be one of the most important restorative material, because of its certain unmatchable properties. It continues to be used as a restorative material because of the following reasons -
• It adapts readily to cavity walls and is easy to insert.
• Little dimensional change occurs during the hardening process.
• The working time is sufficient for placement, condensation, and carving.
• It reaches compressive strengths as high as 80,000 psi, yet it does not wear the opposing tooth structure.
• Marginal microleakage is minimal.
• It endures the harsh oral environment very well.

LIMITATIONS AS RESTORATIVE MATERIAL

However, silver amalgam, as a restorative material, has certain intrinsic limitations, which caused the downfall of this material from the position of undisputed king of restorative materials, which it retained for more than 50 years by virtue of remaining the material of first choice in most of the restorative cases. However, in last few decades, with the invention of certain new materials, its position has been challenged up to great extent, with the Silver amalgam losing its luster as a restorative material. Some of the reasons of its decline are as follows -

• The silver/gray/black color is in sharp contrast to tooth structure and is esthetically undesirable.
• The presence of mercury in the material.

- It may be subject to discoloration/tarnish over time.
- It is non-adhesive and requires sufficient tooth structure support to be retained.
- Its high thermal conductivity requires placement of sufficient base or liner to protect the pulp.

COMPOSITION

The mixing of a metal alloy powder and mercury forms dental amalgam. Mercury is a metal that's liquid at room temperature. The alloy component contains three primary metals—silver, tin, and copper. Most modern dental amalgams are zinc-free and have greater than 12% copper (high copper content).

Mercury

Mercury is only metal that is liquid at room temperature. Any metal mixed with mercury is an "amalgam." It is the mixing of the powdered alloy and mercury that creates the dental amalgam that has been the primary posterior restorative for many years. Dental amalgam is specifically mercury, silver, tin, copper, and any other metals used. Mercury is poisonous and care must be taken in its handling. Pure mercury should have a bright, shiny, silvery, mirror-like surface. If the surface is dull or appears to be contaminated, the mercury should be filtered through a clean cloth. Mercury may be carefully handled in its liquid form because it is not readily absorbed. However, if vaporized by heat, it can be absorbed through the pores of the skin or inhaled and absorbed through the lungs. Almost all dental amalgam today is sold in pre-dose capsules to minimize any handling of mercury. Use a no-touch technique by wearing gloves, a mask, and glasses if you should have to work with mercury or dental amalgams. Mercury spill kits are available to safely clean up any loose, free mercury. These kits contain a powder (such as sulfur) that combines with the liquid mercury to form a compound that can be safely and easily cleaned up. The household vacuum should not be used to clean up mercury spills because it will tend to vaporize the mercury. Mercury vapor has no odor, color, or taste and cannot be easily detected. Polyethylene bags should be used to dispose of any mercury-contaminated items. Proper ventilation in treatment rooms (operatories) is necessary. Air-filter systems need to be checked and/or changed regularly to reduce the possibility of inhaling mercury vapors. Mercury vapor monitors or monitoring equipment is available. However, the use of pre-capsulated amalgams has virtually eliminated the need for them.

AMALGAM RESTORATION PROCEDURES

Dental amalgam has long been the restorative of choice for posterior restorations. It is also used as a core material to prepare a base for a crown or bridge. However, in cases where the darkness of the amalgam might be visible in the patient's smile, dentists are now more frequently choosing the latest in composite resin bonding systems, which closely match the tooth shade of the patient. Another change in the amalgam technique that is becoming popular is called the bonded amalgam.

Cavity Preparation

After viewing the appropriate x-rays to determine the size and probable shape of the decayed or missing tooth structure, the dentist will select the rotary instruments (carbides or diamonds) for use in the high-speed handpiece. The cutting of tooth structure is always done with sufficient water spray as a coolant. The assistant should hold the high-volume evacuator on the opposite side of the tooth to draw the water across the tooth, providing maximum cooling effect. The prepared cavity is then rinsed with a water spray and dried with an air syringe for final assessment. The dentist examines the preparation before staring the restoration step to make sure that-
• All unsound tooth structure has been removed
• The proper retention form has been created
• The preparation is clean and dry.

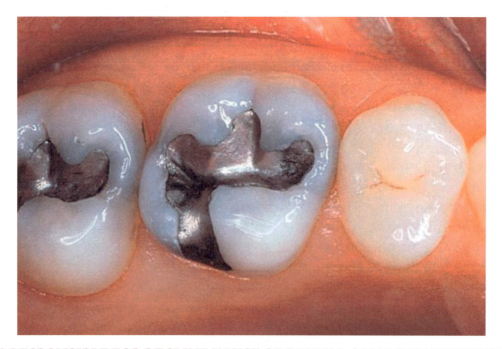

FACTORS RESPONSIBLE FOR DECLINE IN USE OF DENTAL AMALGAM IN RECENT TIME

During past 20 years there has been a continual decrease in the use of amalgam. The decrease is due to numerous factors. Some of the main factors are as follows:

    (I)   Fluoridated water supplies, better oral hygiene, use of sealants & other strategies have significantly reduced dental caries in younger individuals.

    (II)   Amalgam contains mercury that is a health hazard. Dental personals can be exposed to mercury either in the form of vapour or as particulate amalgam dust that can be inhaled from the air.

(III)   Hypersensitivity to amalgam: The production of delayed hypersensitivity, contact reactions on the skin and mucous membrane including lichenoid lesions are reported but are rare.

(IV)   Increased use of esthetic dental materials such as resin composites. The movement away from metallic restorative materials to more tooth-colored materials is understandable and well justified.

POSSIBLE ALTERNATIVES TO AMALGAM

A.   Metal Alloys

a.   Gold Inlays
b.   Gold Foil
c.   Mercury free direct filling alloy
d.   Gallium alloy

B.   Non-Metal/Tooth colored alternative

a.   Glass ionomer cement
b.   Composite resin
c.   Glass ionomer-resin hybrids
d.   Ceramics

From the above-mentioned list of alternatives, it can be very well made out that amalgam is economical and reliable material. It is not dead but its position in dentistry has changed. With the advent of concept of bonding amalgam to tooth structure, a better tomorrow is forecasted. Bonded amalgam offers advantages of conservative preparation.

CHAPTER 14
COMPOSITE RESINS

From their initial introduction in the late 1960s to the present, composites have undergone dramatic evolution, especially with respect to their adaptability, handling, retention, and esthetics. A composite is composed of a resin polymer with a filler of glass, silica, and/or quartz. Similar to a wall composed of mortar and bricks, a composites resin matrix holds the filler particles together. Most composite resin bases are usually BIS-GMA (bisphenol A–glycidyl methacrylate) or urethane dimethacrylate. The filler particles are coated with a silane coupling agent that bonds to the particles and allows the particles to bond to the resin matrix. Composites can be classified according to their process of polymerization initiation and filler type.

POLYMERIZATION
The resin matrix chemically takes its final form through a process called polymerization. In simple terms, we can call it hardening or curing. It's an involved chemical process in which monomers (simple chemical compounds with a single unit) and oligomers (chemical compounds with a few structural units) form long-chain polymers (compounds with repeating structural units). There are three methods by which this polymerization process is initiated.

Self-Cure Composites
The first composites that were introduced in the field of restorative dentistry, were self-cure composites. In this variety of composite, the polymerization cycle starts by mixing two components (labeled base and catalyst, or A and B) and an initiator (a chemical component that begins polymerization, usually a benzoyl peroxide). After the mixing this material sets on its own in 2 to 4 minutes, so the dentist has that much time to place the material before the composite hardens to its final form. Because of its self-curing nature this variety of composites requires quick placement. Considerable time is necessary to finish and polish the very hard final form of the composite. Working time is approximately 1 to 11/2 minutes, with setting time about 4 to 5 minutes from the start of the mix.

Light Cure Composites

To overcome the shortcomings of the self-cure composites and to give the control of setting time in the hands of the user of the material, the researchers have developed composites that polymerize quickly only upon exposure to light of a certain wavelength. These light cure (or photo cure) composites provide the operator more time for placement and require less time for finishing. Unlike the self-cure composites (which have two components that must be mixed), the light cure composites are produced as single-paste formulas with the initiator (usually camphorquinone) included in the paste. A light cure composite can be manipulated until the operator exposes it to a curing light, giving the option to the operator to satisfactorily finish the filling before initiating the polymerization or setting of the material. A curing light is an instrument designed to emit the type of light required to initiate polymerization. When the initiator absorbs the light, polymerization occurs. This hardening can often be achieved with a 20-second exposure to the curing light. When this light curing takes place, be sure to wear your shield and protective glasses and not look directly at the light, as it may harm the eyes.

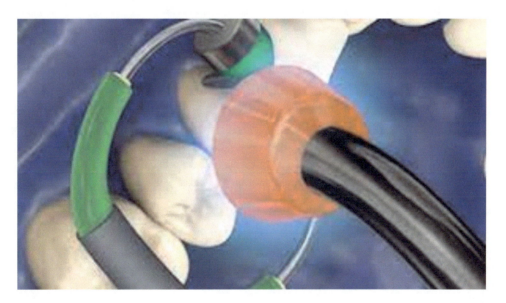

Dual Cure Composites

In certain applications, such as the placement of resin or porcelain inlays, onlays, and veneers or the case of bonded amalgams, it is impossible for the curing light to penetrate through the restorative to polymerize the composite resin cement. A light cured composite cement used in these situations would only polymerize at the exposed margins. Thus, researchers developed the dual cure composites. The dual cure materials contain two initiators - a light cure initiator and a self-cure initiator. The light cure component allows for rapid polymerization of the composite material at the critical margins on exposure to light curing light, while the self-cure initiator ensures that the composite underneath the restorative completes polymerization, without exposure to light source.

FILLER TYPES

There are three categories of filler types based on the size of the particles and their distribution.

Macrofilled Composites

The composites introduced initially used to contain relatively large filler particles of irregularly shaped quartz with a range of 1 to 38 microns in size. These composites were self-cure in nature. These macrofilled composites used to have higher wear and tear resistance because of higher compressive strength. But they used to carry some shortcomings also. Once placed, the large particle size of the macrofill would leave a microscopically rough surface when finished. This surface tended to accumulate stain and plaque or suffer from plucking. Plucking is the process through which the filler particles are removed or lost from the resin matrix. The factors such as expansion, contraction, and the various strains placed by biting and chewing will loosen or knock out the particles. Macrofills are available in self-cure and light cure versions.

Microfilled Composites

The microfilled composites represent the composites with the smallest filler particles. Pure microfills contain filler particles under 1 micron in size, often as small as 0.04 micron. These filler particles are primarily colloidal silica. Smaller filler particles create a smoother composite surface. First introduced as self-cure materials, they are an improvement over the macrofills due to their highly polishable surface. However, they do not have as strong a compressive or shear strength and are subject to fracture or chipping under shear strains. So, there use was generally restricted to anterior teeth or non-stress bearing restorations. Microfills are available in self-cure and light cure versions.

Hybrid Composites

Hybrid composites get their name because they contain more than one type of filler particle. They are the mixture of microfilled and macrofilled composites. Most commonly, they would be a glass particle with a range of 1–3 microns in size and a colloidal silica particle of 0.04 micron in size. When these two particles are combined, the composite reaches optimum strength. Other changes in chemical composition have also improved the handling properties of the hybrids:
• Minimizing the tackiness, or tendency to stick to the placement instrument and pull the material away when the instrument is withdrawn
• Increasing the viscosity for easier packing and shaping
• Eliminating slump and flow, once placed, and maintaining the desired shape
• Changing some formulations so fluoride is released

Hybrid composites match more closely the refractive and reflective light properties of tooth structure. Therefore, they blend in and match the existing tooth's color and characteristics better. Hybrid composites polish much like microfills, resulting in a shiny, smooth surface. The addition of the glass particles makes hybrid composites less likely to fracture and chip because of the increased compressive and shear strengths. Today's most popular hybrid composites are all light cure in nature.

Precautions

• Do not use composites in the presence of eugenol-containing cements or copal varnishes, or with chloroform present. Aromatic medicaments such as eugenol and chloroform will affect the composite's ability to polymerize correctly.

• When using a light cure composite, be sure to keep the fresh composite in its light-protective syringe or compule until its used. Although normal overhead lighting won't properly polymerize the light cure composite, it can affect the handling properties—making the material more difficult to place and manipulate.

• If a patient's gingival tissue is unhealthy, the dentist may postpone treatment until the tissue has improved. Bleeding and moisture contamination will interfere with the setting reaction.

Bonding Systems

The first composites were placed in a similar fashion as the traditional amalgams. The cavity preparation was made with a box form for retention; a calcium hydroxide liner was placed, and the composite restoration was completed. With no direct bonding to the surrounding tooth structure, these composite restorations were susceptible to microleakage. Failure would frequently occur, which lead to the concept of different ways of bonding composites to enamel or dentin.

Enamel is primarily (96%) inorganic, containing mostly hydroxyapatite (a calcium compound). On the other hand, dentin has a higher percentage of organic components. Its 70% inorganic and 30% organic matter (e.g., collagen) and water. This results in drastically different surfaces for an adhesive to bond.

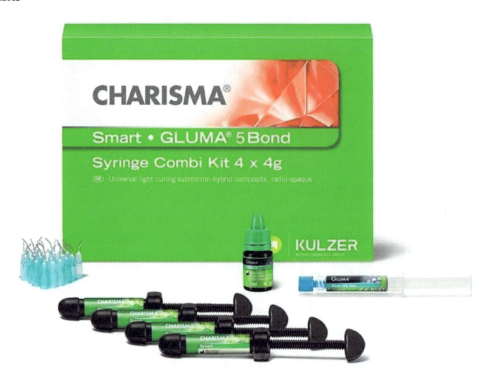

Enamel Bonding

Michael Buonocore of the Eastman Dental Center in Rochester, New York, was the first researcher who brought the concept of Enamel Bonding. His research demonstrated that the enamel rod structure could be opened up with a phosphoric acid etchant. The etchant created a very rough microscopic surface into which the unfilled resins would flow. Upon hardening, the resin provides a mechanical attachment to the tooth. On the basis of his research study the first bonding systems for composites bonded to the enamel of the tooth, was introduced. In this enamel bonding technique 35–50% solution (liquid or gel) of phosphoric acid is used, which is carefully painted over the involved enamel margins of the prepared cavity and it is allowed to remain in contact with enamel surface for 30–60 seconds. In this process, called as acid etching, the acid penetrates into the enamel rods, opening up their prism structures. After that, the acid is rinsed away with water and then the tooth is thoroughly dried, giving a dull or chalky-white appearance to the etched enamel. The enamel bond resin (basically the same resin polymers as in the composite to be used but without any filler particles) is painted over the etched enamel and dentin surfaces, so that the resin flows into the opened prisms and, upon polymerization, forms resin tags. After that, the composite restorative material is placed, which bonds to the enamel bond resin, completing the restoration.

Enamel bonding is, therefore, a mechanical system consisting of the resin tags locked into the etched enamel. The initial types of enamel bonds were low-viscosity, self-cure variety with limited working time. They consisted of two liquid components that were mixed and painted onto the etched enamel.

Subsequently, light cure versions of enamel bond systems were introduced, which consist of a one-component liquid whose polymerization is initiated by a curing light.

The third kind of enamel bonds are the dual cure versions, which consist of two components that can be light cured or will self-cure if the light can't reach the material.

Dentin Bonding

After the success of enamel bonding systems, the dentin bonding material were introduced for the use in composite restorative procedures. It gave the additional bonding and the more reliability to composite restoration procedures.

As the dentin of the tooth is so close to the vital pulpal tissues, care must be taken as to what we treat the dentin with. Modern dentin etchant/conditioners prepare the dentin surface for bonding by removing or modifying the *smear layer.* The smear layer is the layer of the tooth that remains after the drilling or debridement is completed. It consists of attached and loose organic and inorganic matter. Modern dentin primer/adhesives attempt to mechanically lock to the prepared dentin and chemically adhere to the collagen in the dentin.

The technique for dentin bonding is as follows:

1. The preparation is cleaned with a commercially available cavity cleanser/disinfectant, pumice, or chlorhexidine. It's then rinsed thoroughly with a water spray.

2. The entire cavity preparation is then etched or conditioned with the supplied etchant (35% phosphoric acid solution). The enamel is coated first, and then the sensitive dentin is coated. Dentin needs only 15–20 seconds of exposure, while the enamel can be etched for up to 60 seconds.

3. All surfaces are thoroughly rinsed to remove any trace of the etchant. The enamel should be dried to ensure that excess moisture is removed from the newly created prisms. Most new dentin bonding systems have been shown to bond better to moist or damp dentin. Thus, the dentin should be dried only enough to remove excess standing "puddles" of water.

4. The primer (the solution used in dentin bonding) is then placed over the entire cavity preparation. Multiple coats are required by some systems, for which the manufacturer's instructions must be followed. Dentin-bonding primers are typically hydrophilic (water-attractive) monomers that wet the tooth structure and prepare the surfaces for the bonding resin. In almost all systems, the dentin primer is dried from the tooth.

5. The bonding resin is then applied over the primer. Many dentin-bonding resins contain adhesion promoters in addition to their base composition of unfilled resin. These adhesion promoters enhance the resins ability to adhere to the tooth structure. The bonding resin

penetrates into the intertubular and peritubular dentin, forming a complex mixture of tooth structure and resin, which is called the *hybrid layer*. It is this hybrid layer that makes dentin bonding nearly as strong as enamel bonding. Even more importantly, the enhanced seal of the hybrid layer reduces or eliminates microleakage, which has been implicated in causing sensitivity, restorative failure, and recurrent decay. After the application of the bonding and its curing the tooth is restored as usual with the selected composite resin.

Resin Cements

Resin cements are unfilled or slightly filled versions of dental composites. That is, they contain little or no filler particles. As with their composite cousins, the resin is primarily BISGMA (bisphenol A–glycidyl methacrylate) or urethane dimethacrylate. Resin cements are available in the three polymerization types that composites are available: self-cure, light cure, and dual cure.

Self-cure resin cements are used in cases where a light wouldn't reach to initiate polymerization, such as under crowns, bridges, and resin-bonded bridges. Other uses for self-cure resin cements include cementing endodontic posts and bonding orthodontic brackets.

Light cure resin cements can be used in applications where the light will reach the material to initiate the polymerization. For thin anterior veneers and certain porcelain crowns, these resin cements feature special coloration to esthetically match the existing tooth structures.

Dual cure resin cements are the best to use with inlays and onlays, although they could be used in any application resin cement might be used. Dual cure cements are also used in the bonded amalgam technique.

Bonded Amalgams

Adhesive dentistry has evolved to the point that dentin bonding provides the tightest marginal seal available today. For this reason, newer techniques have combined the advantages of this adhesive technology with the long-popular dental amalgam. These new techniques create the bonded amalgam, which is essentially an amalgam restoration placed with the dentin bonding system. It can even be used to repair or add to an older amalgam restoration.

Varnishes

Varnishes are used to protect the tooth from sensitivity due to microleakage and irritants. They are "painted" over all exposed dentin. Upon hardening, they form a seal over the dentinal tubules.

Copal Resins

The original varnish formulations are *copal* (gum) resin-based products and are used under dental amalgams being placed in the traditional technique. Some copal varnishes also include fluoride or antimicrobial agents for enhanced protection should microleakage occur. The copal resin is carried in a solvent of ether or chloroform. The solvent rapidly evaporates, leaving the resin behind.

Polyamide Resins

When dental composites became popular, it was found that the copal varnishes interfered with the composite's cure. Because of this interference, a new generation of varnishes based on polyamide resins was developed. This polyamide layer provides the same properties as the copal resin layer, while maintaining full compatibility with the composite resins. However, varnishes are no longer used with composite resins.

CHAPTER 15
CAVITY PREPARATION

Cavity Preparation Types

Cavity preparations are named for the tooth surfaces involved. Compound names are created as for line angles. For example, a common three-surface posterior restoration involving the mesial, distal, and occlusal tooth surfaces is designated MOD and spelled mesio-occluso-distal.

Classification of Cavities

There are five classifications of cavities according to Black's description.

• **Class I** cavities are pit and fissure decay that involve the occlusal, buccal, or lingual surfaces of a posterior tooth Class I caries may also be lingual surfaces of maxillary incisors.

• **Class II** cavities involve the proximal surface of posterior teeth, such as the mesial and distal surfaces. In the cavity design, the occlusal is usually included.

• **Class III** cavities are found on the proximal surfaces of anterior teeth but do not involve the incisal edge. In the cavity design, the lingual or facial surfaces are usually included.

• **Class IV** cavities are found on the proximal surfaces of anterior teeth that involve the incisal edge.

• **Class V** cavities are found on the gingival third of the labial, buccal, or lingual surfaces of any tooth. This can include root erosion/abrasion.

A sixth classification of cavities, **Class VI**, was added to Black's classifications. These cavities involve the incisal edge of anterior teeth and/or the cuspal tips of posterior teeth.

CHAPTER 16
RADIATION HAZARDS

R adiobiology is the study of the effects of radiation on the tissues and organs of the body. Naturally occurring radiation is uncontrollable and can be found all around us in the form of the sun and minerals such as uranium and radium. In contrast, man-made production of x-radiation is controlled in the x-ray machine.

The dentist and his or her staff should know how to protect the public as well as themselves from overexposure. When you work with your patients, obey the safety precautions you have learned every time you expose a radiograph. The principle "as little as reasonably achievable" (ALARA) has been adopted as a rule of thumb for maintaining radiation safety. Only the proper amount of radiation needed to produce a diagnostic quality radiograph should be used, and only those areas necessary should be radiographed.

Over the past 50 years, there have been many advances in three areas that have affected dental radiology:
1. Research into the effects of overexposure to radiation
2. Development of more modern x-ray machines capable of reducing the amount of radiation exposure but still giving a good diagnostic radiograph
3. Better education of radiation workers.

RADIATION HAZARDS
Dental radiographs are considered specific area radiographs as they are taken of small areas and not the whole body. There is no absolutely safe dose of radiation; any amount causes damage. The amount of radiation received affects the severity of the damage done—the higher the dose, the more damage. The effects of radiation are cumulative. Today's effect is added to yesterday's effect, and tomorrow's effect will be added to today's effect, and so forth throughout life. Overexposure to radiation is known to be a consistent cause of cancer. Naturally occurring radiation exposure is added to medical/dental exposure.

All radiations are ionizing in nature. All cells in body grow and divide, forming new cells.

When a change happens, the cells work together over time to bring everything back into balance. Ionizing radiation breaks the cell bonds and disturbs the balance of the cell. In an effort to regain normalcy, atoms combine with other disturbed atoms, thereby forming a new substance. This substance may be harmful to the cell or organ that was struck by the x-rays. The amount of damage that has done is directly related to two factors: the time in the life of the cell that exposure occurs, and the type of cell or tissue involved in the exposure.

The most sensitive time for a cell is when it's dividing to form two new cells. This cell division is called mitosis. More damage is done to the cell if it is irradiated during mitosis. The type of tissue involved in the exposure is important because each cell has a different rate of mitosis. Radiosensitive and radioresistant are the terms used to describe the degree of sensitivity each type of tissue has. Tissues that have a fast rate of reproduction are said to be radiosensitive, or more sensitive to radiation. Those that have a slower rate of change are said to be radioresistant, or more resistant to damage. Cells that reproduce rapidly, such as the human embryo and reproductive cells, are most radiosensitive and least radioresistant. Cells that do not change very much after they've fully formed, such as enamel or bone cells, are least radiosensitive and most radioresistant.

Radiation has two effects on tissue or cells: the direct effect and the indirect effect. The direct effect occurs when the nucleus of the cell is directly hit by radiation. The cell dies immediately, or at the time of mitosis. In the treatment of cancer, the aim of radiation is to have a direct effect on the cancer cells, so they die quickly before spreading. The indirect effect occurs when cells are changed in a destructive manner. This often occurs in the case of the reproductive cells. Unfortunately, damage may not be evident for a long time. The number of cells indirectly affected or killed determines the amount of damage done and how much the function of the cells or organ is altered.

Radiation effects can be somatic or genetic. Somatic effects are seen in all areas of the body except in the genetic tissue. Remember, radiation effects accumulate in the body. The first signs of radiation illness are changes in the blood. For changes in the blood to occur, the entire body would have to be overexposed to radiation. It would take a large dose at one time for this to occur. Dental x-rays cover specific small areas. The whole body is not directly exposed, and the dental machine is not capable of producing the amount of radiation necessary for somatic effects.

Genetic effects include damage done to reproductive cells that can be passed on and may not be evident for several generations. For this reason, it is important to follow all the safety measures and never overexpose your patients or yourself to radiation.

Effects of overexposure are short term or long term. Short-term effects occur with high doses of radiation over a short period of time, such as in cancer therapy. The long-term effects occur with both high doses over a short term and small doses over a long term. Genetic diseases are the effect of small doses over a long term. The radiation worker must be protected from small doses over a long period of time.

STAGES OF EFFECT OF RADIATION EXPOSURE

There are three stages of radiation effects:

1. **Latent period**—It is the period from the time of exposure until the effect is seen. The first sign of overexposure to radiation is erythema or redness of the skin.

2. **Short-term effects**—Seen within a week of exposure.

3. **Long-term effects**—Seen in years or decades or even in the next generation.

The effects of radiation on cells are cumulative. Whatever damage is done during a first exposure is added to damage from the next exposure, and so on. If exposures are extensive (cover a large area) and not much time passes between exposures, the cells do not have time to correct themselves. In the case of the cancerous tumor, this is good because it is eventually destroyed. If good tissue around the tumor is also destroyed, it is not good. The destruction of tissue is both the benefit and hazard of radiation.

Between exposures, the body tries to return to normal. Seventy-five percent of the cell damage is repaired within 24 hours. Repair continues over time at this same rate. So, on the first day, 75 percent of the whole damage is repaired; on the second day, 75 percent of the remaining 25 percent of damage is repaired; and by the third day, 75 percent of the remaining 6.25 percent of damage is repaired; and so on. This is assuming that the cells are not subjected to more radiation. There have been no incidents reported about radiation injuries caused by dental x-rays. There are always minor risks, but the information gained in the diagnosis of dental disease or even medical conditions in oral tissues far outweighs the risks. Today, better equipment and other innovations allow very little radiation exposure.

MEASUREMENTS OF RADIATION EXPOSURE

Several different terms are used to measure ionizing radiation. Researchers have defined a unit of radiation exposure as 1 roentgen, or 1 R. One R involves the scientific measurement of the amount of x-radiation required to change a very tiny amount of air at standard conditions of temperature and pressure. A unit of radiation that enters the body is called a radiation absorbed dose (rad). The effect of that unit on the body is called relative biological effect (RBE). Scientists combined these measurements to describe the roentgen equivalent in man (rem), which is the physical and biological effect of various amounts of radiation on tissue. Using rem measurement, scientists have been able to adopt a maximum permissible dose (MPD) for the purpose of radiation safety.

The National Council on Radiation Protection and Measurements (NCRPM) in the North America and similar organizations in most of other countries, have established limits on how much radiation an operator can be exposed to. The recommended limits are 0.3 R per week, 3.0 R per 13-week period, and 5.0 R per year.

The Radiation Protection Bureau of Canada is responsible for delivering Health Canada's environmental and occupational radiation protection program. The Radiation Health Assessment Division (RHAD) contributes assessments and guidance to help Canadians reduce and manage risks from ionizing radiation exposure. The National Dose Registry (NDR) runs Canada's national database for occupational exposure to ionizing radiation. The NDR collects and maintains dose information about Canadian workers to ensure that life-long records are available to individuals, and to support provincial and federal regulatory requirements for managing exposure. The NDR issues summary reports on occupational exposure in Canada and participates in epidemiological studies, solely or in collaboration with other agencies, to generate information on the assessment and management of risk from occupational exposure.

Dental offices or hospital are supposed to provide all the auxiliary staff involved with radiology process, a monitoring badge called Dosimeter badge, which measures any exposure to x-rays so that the limits will not be exceeded. The badges are collected every 13 weeks and sent to a radiology laboratory for processing, and then a report is sent back. If there is any evidence of exposure, corrective measures in radiation safety techniques should be taken. Equipment should also be inspected to see if there is a leak in the area of the machine where radiation is produced.

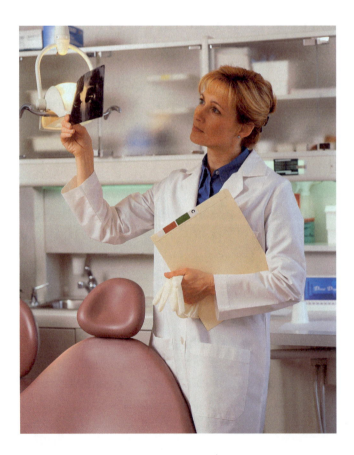

RADIATION SAFETY

Manufacturers built safety measures into the modern x-ray machines. These include aluminum filters and a lead lining, which are used to absorb rays that could harm tissue. A lead shield is also added to the x-rays films. Older units should be inspected to be sure there are no leaks in the tube head or elsewhere.

In addition of the above-mentioned safety measures, some precautions taken while exposing the radiographs can restrict the amount of Radiation harm for both the patients and the operator.

PROTECTING THE X-RAY MACHINE OPERATOR

- Never hold the film in the patient's mouth.
- Never stand in the path of the primary beam used to take the radiograph.
- Stand six feet behind the tube head, behind a lead screen, or out of the room.
- Have equipment inspected regularly.
- Wear a monitoring badge (Dosimeter Badge).

SAFETY MEASURES TO PROTECT THE PATIENT FROM RADIATION

Sufficient protection of the patient from the radiation hazards is also of great importance in modern dental offices. Some of the safety measures, which should be followed in all the dental offices, while exposing the patients to X-radiation, during the process of taking the radiographs, are as follows:

- Use of a lead apron with a cervical collar.
- Ask the patient about any recent medical radiation therapy.
- Make sure that unnecessary radiographs aren't being taken.
- Use of high-speed film.

CHAPTER 17
DENTAL RADIOGRAPHS

TYPES OF RADIOGRAPHS

Radiographs are intraoral or extraoral. The Bite-wing (BW), periapical (PA), and occlusal (Occ) radiographs are examples of intraoral radiographs. The extraoral radiographs are the panoramic and cephalometric (cephalogram) radiographs.

INTRAORAL RADIOGRAPHS

(1) Bite-wing radiographs. Bite-wings are taken of posterior teeth usually to check for any interproximal caries or periodontal condition.

A bite-wing radiograph must show the crown areas of the upper and lower posterior teeth from the mesial of the first premolars to the distal of the third molars.

The dentist can use these to diagnose
• Interproximal decay—Decay between the mesial and distal areas which cannot be seen or felt with the explorer.

• Restoration contour—Overhang of silver or composite filling material, which is usually under the gingival tissue. Extra filling material left at the margin of the cavity can cause irritation to the tissue and act as a food trap.

• Pulp size in relation to caries

• Bone levels around the teeth—Bite-wings detect the beginnings of periodontal bone loss.

• The location of subgingival calculus.

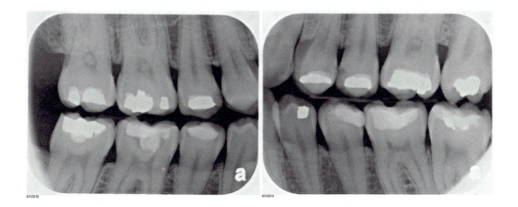

(2) Periapical (PA) radiographs. The periapical radiograph is taken to get the image of the root, crown, apex, surrounding bone and periodontal ligament support of an individual tooth and problems, such as an apical abscess, broken root, or other painful emergencies. One periapical film may show three or four teeth, depending on size. The tooth that is to be examined should be centered in the film.

(3) Occlusal radiographs. The occlusal radiograph is taken to show:
· The position of permanent dentition under the deciduous teeth
· Destruction of tissue from a palatal or sublingual pathology
· Fractures
· Size of the dental arches
· Mandibular tori (an overgrowth of bone found on the lingual surface of the mandibular bone)
· The condition of an edentulous (without natural teeth) ridge

FULL MOUTH SURVEY (FMX)
 The full mouth survey consists of 14 to 19 individual radiographs, depending on the size of the radiograph used for anterior radiographs and if bite-wings are also taken. There are several different sizes of intraoral radiographs, which are used for different purposes.

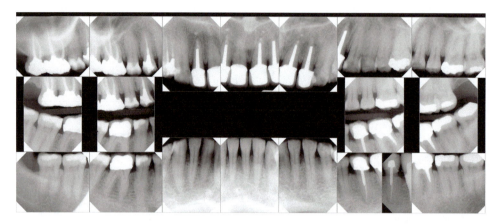

For FMX generally the following pattern is followed so that no area is missed or double exposed:

• Anterior—6 Periapical radiographs having three maxillary and three mandibular
• Bite-wings—4 radiographs with two on each side
• Posterior—8 radiographs with two maxillary right, two mandibular right, two maxillary left and two mandibular left

This series is only taken if the doctor feels overall conditions in the patient's mouth need a more complete examination than is possible with a mirror and explorer.

EXTRAORAL RADIOGRAPHS

(1) **Panoramic radiographs.** They show the entire dentition and surrounding tissues and structures on one radiograph The Panorex and Panelipse radiographs are types of panoramic radiographs taken as overall surveys of the jaws.

These radiographs are taken to diagnose

➢ Pathology in tissue (growths or abnormal bone)
➢ Development of permanent dentition under deciduous
➢ Position of impacted teeth
➢ Jaw fractures
➢ Location of foreign bodies (objects imbedded in tissue)
➢ Abnormalities of the temporomandibular joint (TMJ), the hinge joint of the lower jaw
➢ Relationship of one jaw to the other

The extraoral radiographs are used mostly by oral surgeons and orthodontists to diagnose the areas which relate to their treatment. General dentists can use them as an aid to identify problems which may need the further attention. However, these exposures don't give the sharp image of individual teeth needed to diagnose caries or the detailed conditions shown in bite-wing and periapical radiographs.

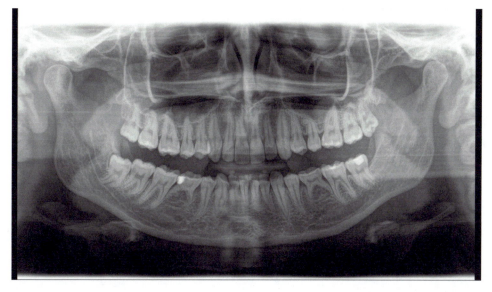

(2) Cephalometric radiographs. The cephalometric (or cephalogram) radiograph is taken of the skull in the frontal or lateral view.

The cephalogram is used to

• Obtain measurements for prosthetics or orthodontics

• See abnormal conditions in the head and face structures

• See TMJ problems

• Locate pathology

• Locate fractures

• See abnormal development of the relationship between the upper and lower jaw

(3) Water's projection. Another type of extraoral radiograph used mostly by specialists is called the Water's projection. It is taken of the maxillary and frontal sinus areas to find the extent of a sinus condition or infection.

NEW IMAGING TECHNIQUES

Xeroradiography

New technology has brought new ways to examine oral tissues and the teeth. Xeroradiography is a new method of recording x-ray images on an electrically charged plate (not film). It combines x-ray exposure with the same technology used in the office copy machines to produce a photographic image rather than the transparent radiograph. No darkroom processing is needed.

Radiovisiography (RVG)

This method uses a sensor placed in the mouth to project the x-ray image onto a computer screen. It can then enlarge the image or any part of it and print out a picture for patient education, record, and for diagnostic and treatment planning. The images taken so can also be stored on computer hardware.

MRI

Nuclear magnetic resonance (NMR) imaging (also known as MRI) is used in medicine to show slices of body tissues, bones, and the brain without the use of x-radiation. It is being studied for possible application in dentistry.

Though exposure to x-radiation is being reduced in some of these new methods, the technology is very expensive.

CHAPTER 18

ENDODONTIC TERMINOLOGY AND CONDITIONS

E ndodontics is the field of dentistry concerned with the biology and pathology of the dental pulp and periapical tissues. The high degree of success with the various endodontic methods is largely responsible for the modern dentist's claim that extractions are almost never necessary.

Anatomy of the Pulp Cavity

A healthy tooth has a hollow canal within the hard layers of enamel, cementum, and dentin. This passageway consists of the root canal in the root portion and the pulp chamber within the crown of the tooth. The root canal and the pulp chamber of a healthy tooth are filled with a soft, highly sensitive, highly vascular tissue called the pulp. The pulp is important during the formation of the tooth, but it can also be very troublesome later on.

INDICATIONS AND CONTRAINDICATIONS FOR ENDODONTIC TREATMENT

Indications

The major indications for root canal therapy are if the pulp has an irreversible pulpitis or is necrotic. These conditions may be determined by the sensitivity of the tooth, pain on chewing or percussion, or the presence of a periapical radiolucency as seen on a radiograph of the tooth. While these criteria are used to determine whether or not endodontic therapy is warranted, other considerations must be kept in mind.

Contraindications

The following are examples of contraindications to endodontic therapy:
• The tooth in question is unrestorable.
• The canals cannot be negotiated
• There is a perforation of the root or pulp chamber either by caries or mechanical means.
• Internal or external root resorption is present.
• A severe periodontal condition exists that may cause eventual tooth loss on its own.

ENDODONTIC CONDITIONS

PULPITIS

The pulp is made up of complex connective tissue. It contains blood vessels, connective tissue fibers, various types of cells, and nerves. Exposed pulp tissue is quite sensitive to touch and irritation. Usually in response of any type of irritation the pulpal cells get inflamed, which can be extremely painful. This condition is called pulpitis.

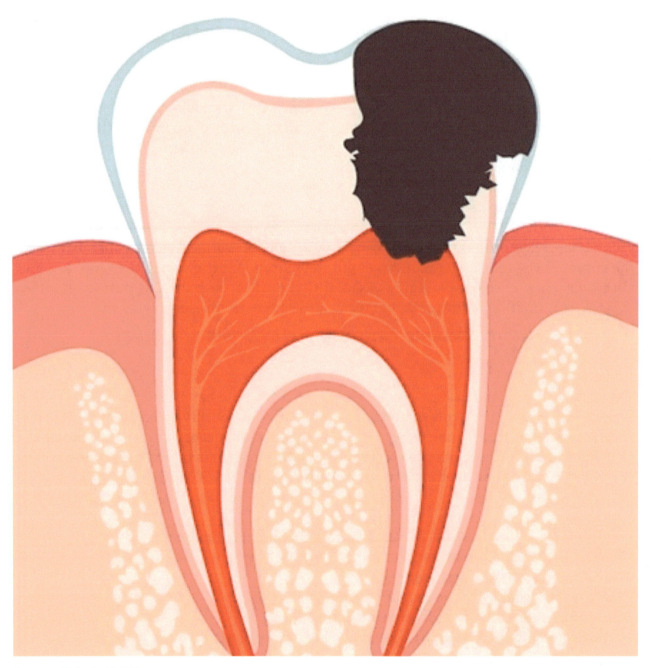

Reversible Pulpitis:

Reversible pulpitis responds with short duration pain upon thermal (hot or cold) stimulation and returns to normal almost immediately. It isn't a situation that requires the removal of inflamed pulpal tissue and root canal therapy. Removal of the etiologic factors, such as caries or faulty restorations, is the treatment of choice. Once the cause is removed, the inflammatory process reverses itself and the tooth becomes asymptomatic.

Irreversible Pulpitis:

Irreversible pulpitis is characterized by a long and painful response to thermal stimulation that does not go away quickly. The pulp of the tooth has an inflammatory process that will not reverse itself. Endodontic therapy is always necessary in the treatment of irreversible pulpitis. The only alternative treatment is extraction of the tooth. A reversible pulpitis can be a stage in the development of irreversible pulpitis, which is more than a mere irritation.

Necrotic Pulp:

The last phase of the pulpal pain process is pulp inflammation leading to complete necrosis (tissue death). At this stage, the patient may have severe pain of a more constant nature along with periradicular (around the root) pain symptoms. The tooth is sensitive to palpation and percussion but has no thermal response or response to the electric pulp tester. A necrotic pulp must be treated by root canal therapy.

Caries-Induced Pulpitis:

Dental caries is the best-known cause of pulpitis. If untreated, dental caries continues its course toward the pulp. As the decay advances, the pulp retreats from the oncoming caries by putting down layers of secondary or reparative dentin, effectively increasing the amount of sound tooth that the decay must destroy before reaching the pulp. Bacteria actually progress ahead of the caries through the dentinal tubules. If remain untreated for long time the caries penetrates into the pulp chamber or root canal, infecting the pulp.

Cellulitis:

The pulpal infection that spreads through the hole in the root end into the surrounding bone may cause generalized swelling of the surrounding gum and soft tissues. This leads to a dangerous inflammatory condition called cellulitis, which, if untreated, can have serious consequences.

Fistula:

Caries-induced pulpitis does not always lead to cellulitis. More often, drainage is innocently established by way of a fistula, which is a tunnel-like opening in the tissue. The common gum boil is a stage in the development of the fistula.

Trauma-Induced Pulpitis:

There are other causes of pulpitis besides caries. Any severe trauma can cause irreversible damage to the pulp and start it on its way to pulpitis. This path may include a stage of chronic pulpitis that lasts for many years before irreversible pulpitis finally develops. Any of the following situations can traumatize the pulp so severely that years later a pulpitis may

develop:
• A physical blow
• Overheating caused by extensive use of a dental drill without proper water coolant
• Unsuccessful partial endodontic procedures such as pulp capping or pulpotomy
• Deep decay apparently successfully treated

Periodontal-Disease-Induced Pulpitis:
Severe periodontal disease can also lead to an infected pulp. When bone has been lost to the level of the apex of one of the roots of a multirooted tooth, periodontal infection may enter the tooth through the apical foramen and attack the pulp from this "backward" direction. This may also occur through accessory canals commonly found in the furcations of molars and along the root surface.

Traumatic Occlusion:
Constant trauma, usually in the form of bruxism (unconscious grinding or clenching of teeth), is another factor to consider in the failure of periapical repair. The most frequently encountered trauma, however, is related to a restoration upon which the patient cannot close without traumatizing the involved tooth. Each restoration of a pulpless tooth should be thoroughly checked for hyperocclusion that could lead to trauma.

Incomplete Fracture:
Fractures of the crown or root (whether complete or incomplete) allow bacterial infection of the pulp. If undetected or untreated, such fractures will result in infection to the pulp and inevitable pulp death.

CHAPTER 19

ROLE OF NUTRITION IN DENTISTRY

As research increasingly suggests a connection between oral health and systemic health, it becomes more important that dental professionals work as part of an interdisciplinary health care team to provide brief nutrition messages to their patients.

It is no wonder that dental professionals feel inadequate when it comes to providing nutrition counseling, after all nutrition receives little time in the dental or dental hygiene curriculum. However, dental professionals can provide some very basic nutrition counseling. All the dental office staff members, interacting with the patient in the operatory, need to maintain current knowledge of nutrition recommendations such as the Dietary Guidelines for patients as they relate to general and oral health and disease. The staff should be well aware and knowledgeable to effectively educate and counsel their patients about proper nutrition and oral health.

It is important for the dental office staff to understand the general nutrition requirements and apply this information to everyday dental practice.
The dental professionals should be able to:
- ➢ Apply the most up-to-date nutrition information to their patient's oral health.
- ➢ Recognize the importance of nutrition to the development, healing, and maintenance of the oral hard and soft tissues.
- ➢ Provide the patients with practical nutrition recommendations.
- ➢ Provide patients with brief nutrition interventions as part of a comprehensive prevention program.

BASIC DENTAL NUTRITION OVERVIEW
Nutrition or diet has effects on oral health by two means:

(1) LOCALIZED EFFECTS
This is the effect we think of most often in dentistry. This refers to the cariogenic (caries promoting) potential of a food that is eaten by a patient. These foods consist of carbohydrates which are broken down by the salivary amylase in the mouth to sucrose, glucose, and fructose which can then be used by the bacterial plaque. The by-product of

the bacterial use of carbohydrates for energy is the production of acid. The acid lowers the pH of the mouth to the critical pH of 5.5 or below which leads to demineralization of the tooth. In a normal, healthy person, this acidic pH lasts for 20 to 30 minutes after eating a fermentable carbohydrate. A common misconception is that we only need to be concerned with the simple sugars eaten when in fact refined, baked starches such as potato chips have actually been found to be highly cariogenic because of their retention on the tooth surfaces.

Unfortunately, dental professionals tend to focus on prevention primarily through improved plaque removal without addressing the other factors involved in caries. Determining which dietary factors may be involved in a patient's caries rate is as important as removing the bacterial plaque. More attention needs to be paid to fluoride to harden the tooth against demineralization as well as assist in remineralization for people of all ages, but in particular for adults.

(2) SYSTEMIC EFFECTS

Nutrients available systemically will impact overall development, growth, and maintenance of the tooth structure, connective tissue, alveolar bone, and oral mucosa. The cells of the oral mucosa turnover every three to seven days. Rapidly growing cells need an adequate supply of all essential nutrients. This makes the oral cavity one of the most sensitive indicators of adequate nutritional status.

Evidence is accumulating to indicate that there is a correlation between systemic osteoporosis, alveolar bone loss, and ultimately tooth loss in post-menopausal women. In a recent prospective study, postmenopausal women who lost teeth were also losing bone mineral of the whole body and femoral neck at greater rates than those who retained their teeth. The rates of change in bone mineral density were significant predictors of tooth loss.

Nutrition is a critical determinant of immune response. Epidemiologic and clinical data suggest that nutritional deficiencies alter immunocompetence and increase the risk of infection in the body, including the oral cavity.

CHAPTER 20

DENTISTRY AND AGE-RELATED DIETARY FACTORS

Although caries control cannot rely solely on dietary interventions, dietary factors must be modified to reduce the risk of caries. Dietary recommendations for caries prevention need to cover the following dietary factors:

(1) Frequency of eating meals and snacks

(2) Oral retentiveness of foods

(3) Length of interval between eating events

(4) Sequence of food consumption

(5) Amount of fermentable carbohydrate consumed

(6) Sugar concentration of the food or drink item

(7) Physical form of the carbohydrate

(8) Proximity of eating to bedtime

CHANGES AND RELATION OF NUTRITIONAL AND DENTAL REQUIREMENTS IN LIFE CYCLE

During the life cycle a number of vulnerable periods, as well as conditions and diseases, occurs that give rise to special oral health risks or nutritional needs. The dental professionals should be aware to identify patients at high nutritional and oral health risk in order to provide early intervention.

(1) PREGNANCY

Many pregnant women suffer significant nausea and vomiting early in the first trimester, which may result in an increase in decay. The repeated vomiting exposes the teeth to gastric acid, and this causes enamel demineralization. Some experts feel brushing should immediately follow a vomiting incident, while others feel that brushing in the presence of increased acidity will enhance the enamel destruction. If vomiting occurs frequently during pregnancy, the patient can be told to rinse immediately after vomiting with sodium bicarbonate to neutralize the gastric acid. The traditional dietary recommendations for nausea are to nibble on soda crackers and dry cereal; however, both are highly retentive fermentable carbohydrates. Oral hygiene procedures may also cause nausea in some pregnant women. Brushing with a child's size toothbrush using only water, followed by fluoride rinses, helps some.

Pregnant women often have cravings for high carbohydrate type foods. They should be encouraged to choose healthy snacks.

Dietary Recommendations:
(I) Less cariogenic snacks such as fresh fruit, vegetables, and dairy products should be encouraged as soon as the nausea has passed

(II) Encourage healthy snacks like yogurt, cheese, popcorn, fruit, and vegetables for pregnancy cravings

(III) If she feels she must have crackers, try to brush after eating them to remove the retained food from her teeth

(2) INFANTS AND CHILDREN
During infancy and early childhood systemic and local factors can affect tooth development and health of both the primary and permanent teeth. Children with special needs are a group at high risk for oral health problems.

Early Childhood Caries
The biggest dental nutrition concern for infants and young children is in preventing early childhood caries. This condition has been called many things over the years including, nursing bottle caries, baby bottle tooth decay (BBTD), nursing caries, and milk bottle syndrome. 20% of children are at high risk for early childhood caries. Infants and children should never be put to bed with a bottle containing anything other than water. Infants, as young as six months, can begin to learn to drink from a cup. By one year, the infant should be weaned from a bottle to a cup. Dental professionals can help to educate pregnant women before children are born on appropriate use of the bottle.

Special Needs Children

(I) Failure to Thrive (FTT)
Parents of the FTT child often feed them very frequently, sometimes as often as every two hours, in an attempt to provide adequate nutrition to meet their needs. The rich carbohydrate diet with higher frequency of intake, make these patients more susceptible to dental caries.

(II) Developmental Delayed Children
Developmentally delayed children have the greatest variation in needs both nutritionally and dentally. These children may have enamel hypoplasia due to medications, fevers, and other medical and congenital conditions. This places them at increased risk of caries; the use of systemic and topical fluorides is helpful in many of such children. Developmental delayed children often have oral sensitivity.

Some special needs children with developmental delays continue to bottle feed because of delays in learning to chew, spoon feed, and eat independently. These children may require a long period of time to eat resulting in an increased length of time the teeth are exposed to cariogenic foods. Often medications used by children are in sucrose-sweetened syrups; these may increase the risk of caries and also cause dry mouth, which further increases caries risk.

The special needs child requires intensive preventive dental therapy with frequent prophylaxis, through home care by parents, and the use of systemic and topical fluorides.

(3) TEENAGERS

80% of an individual's average caries incidence occurs during the teen years. This is an important time to instill preventive nutrition and dental routines to prevent caries. Yet, adolescence is a time of change for young people when they begin to exert their newfound independence in many ways including choosing the foods they eat, and whether to brush or floss their teeth. They often choose foods low in vitamins, and high in fat and sugar. Teen meals are irregular and frequently consist of fast foods and ready-to-eat snack foods high in fermentable carbohydrates.

Eating Disorders

Eating disorders are one of the most prevalent psychiatric/behavior disturbances affecting adolescents. There is a spectrum of eating disorders, which include anorexia nervosa, bulimia nervosa, and binge eating disorder. These are quite complex and require a multidisciplinary team to manage. They often occur in the adolescent and young adult who is struggling with his or her changing body image. The dentist or dental hygienist may be the first to recognize the oral manifestations of an eating disorder. The dental team may be instrumental in linking the patient suffering from eating disorders with needed medical intervention.

(I) Anorexia Nervosa

These patients may have angular cheilitis due to multiple nutrient deficiencies as well as from dehydration of the skin and mucous membranes. There may also be parotid gland dysfunction resulting in xerostomia or dry mouth, which in turn may result in an increased incidence of decay. Approximately 50% of anorexia nervosa patients also practice bulimia, so the dental erosions normally seen in bulimics who practice self-induced vomiting may also be seen in anorexia.

(II) Bulimia Nervosa

Many more oral manifestations are seen in the patient with bulimia because of the recurrent self-induced vomiting that characterizes the condition. These patients indulge in binging behaviors eating large quantities of high calorie, carbohydrate-rich foods over short periods of time. Average intake of food during a binge-eating episode is 3,400 calories over an hour. Purging either by self-induced vomiting, using laxatives, diuretics, restrictive dieting, or vigorous exercise usually follows the binge-eating episode.

The dental complaint that usually brings these patients to the dental office is "sensitive teeth". This results from the chronic exposure of the tooth to gastric acids during vomiting. The classic oral manifestation is enamel erosion on the lingual surfaces of the maxillary anterior teeth. These patients often have a callous or scar near the first knuckle of the index finger from inducing vomiting by sticking the finger down the throat. The object used to cause vomiting may inflict traumatic palatal injuries or bruising. There may also be xerostomia in these patients due to dehydration from vomiting and laxative use. Caries is also a problem, one study indicated a 29% increase in caries rate among this population because of the large amounts of fermentable carbohydrates eaten during binges, vomiting, and xerostomia. The severity of the caries will depend on the frequency of binges, the cariogenicity of the diet, and oral hygiene practices. Brushing immediately after vomiting is not recommended. Instead, advise rinsing with sodium bicarbonate to neutralize the gastric acid after vomiting. After initiating medical intervention, the dental team will need to begin intensive preventive oral hygiene routines to prevent caries.

(III) Binge Eating Disorder (BED)
BED is characterized by the binge eating behaviors in the bulimic patient, but there is no purging either by vomiting, diuretic, or laxative use. This patient is often overweight or obese. The main oral health concern in these patients is the high risk of caries due to the frequent exposure to fermentable carbohydrates.

(4) ADULTS
With the increase of obesity in our society, the incidence and prevalence of chronic diseases is increasing. This development has many implications for nutrition and the management of dental diseases. Other chronic diseases including cancer and gastrointestinal problems have nutritional and oral health connotations as well. The many medications used to treat these conditions also affect the nutrition and oral health status of these patients.

(I) Diabetes Mellitus
Probably the most common chronic disease seen in dental offices is Type 2 Diabetes Mellitus (or Non-Insulin Dependent Diabetes Mellitus-NIDDM). Patients with diabetes are at high risk for periodontal disease, and they also exhibit impaired wound healing.

(II) Drug/Nutrient Interactions
As now a days the dental patients are taking more and more medications. Some medications increase the need for certain nutrients or interfere with their absorption. Of even more concern is the number of medications that cause xerostomia as a side effect of use, which results in an increased caries risk.

(III) Cancer
As medical science advances, patients with cancer are living longer and often undergoing multiple types of treatment. These cancer therapies often have considerable impact on the oral cavity which also affects their nutritional habits.

(5) ELDERLY

The term "elderly" has been traditionally used for those persons who are above 65 years of age. The physiologic changes observed in aging among the healthy elderly that may affect oral health and nutrition are sensory changes, gastrointestinal changes, and immune system alterations. Many elderly persons also suffer from multiple chronic diseases and take multiple medications for these conditions, which in turn more likely to cause xerostomia and place the elderly at increased risk for root caries.

Over 95% of people 65 and older have some loss of periodontal attachment. Moderate to severe periodontal disease, over time, results in gingival recession and exposure of the root surface, which is more susceptible to caries. Loss of the caries protective qualities and immunologic functions of the saliva contribute to the increase in periodontitis and caries incidence.

Dietary Recommendations:
- ➢ Carry a water bottle to sip on to help relieve dry mouth.
- ➢ Use sugar-free breath mints or candies to stimulate saliva

CHAPTER 21
LATEST TRENDS IN DENTISTRY

RADIOVISIOGRAPHY(RVG)

One can come across a customary scenario at a Dental Clinic-a patient approaches a clinic, writhing in toothache, with a gloomy face after spending a painful night. After long time of wait in reception room, eventually gets access to the doctor, who after examining the patient, establishes a provisional diagnosis of his or her condition and announces-need for an x-ray. Patient agrees. X-ray or x-rays taken. But not all the clinics provide the report of x rays instantly as obtaining the x ray report means a trip down the hall to the developing room, a few minutes of developing, processing and drying. In case of failed x-ray image, again the entire procedure has to be repeated. Needless to mention, the patient is provided the next appointment, only to have more prolonged management, further adding to his or her woes.

This familiar scenario has become a memory of past with the invention of Digital Radiographic technology and the electronic readout devices. The current advances in the field of Dentistry are the testimony that the Digital Imaging System is fast replacing and surpassed by the traditional x-ray system with the new, state of the art Dental Digital radiography Techniques. With the advent of this new technology (RadioVisioGraphy), instead of the time consuming and cumbersome procedures of obtaining, developing, and processing of x ray films; dentist and patient can relax and watch the images of teeth and gums right in front on a computer monitor within seconds after the device (Electronic Sensor) is inserted into the patient's mouth.

Various computer-based imaging systems are available today to get the Digital Dental Images by both the direct and indirect ways. In the direct method, a digital electronic sensor is used whereas in the indirect method, imaging plates of various sizes are used in the place of x-ray films. Digital Dental Radiography is a computerized radiographic technic in which an electronic sensor is utilized in lieu of conventional x-ray film. Thus, obtained images are transformed into its digital form and can be viewed into its digital form on the computer monitor. In this technic, electronic sensor is sensitive to x-rays. Hence, when exposed to radiation, it captures the image of an object and sends the electronic message through the fibreoptic cable to the hardware of CPU of computer, which in turn works on it and converts the message obtained into the digital image with the help of software. Digital images so received can be viewed on the computer monitor, which can be worked on and stored in the computer for the permanent record. The main important facet of this technology is the avoidance of x-rays, which are otherwise mandatory to arrive at a proper and final diagnosis and appropriate management planning in any case.

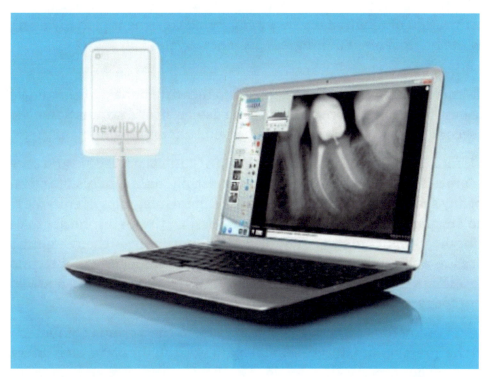

Apart from conserving time of the doctor, his assistant, and the patient by obtaining the quickest scanned images, the other advantages of the technology are too many to mention a few. The prime one among all of them is approximately 90% reduction in x-ray dosage, the doctor and patient used to receive in the conventional x-ray technic. Here they are exposed to only 1/10th of the x-ray dosage delivered in normal conventional x-ray technique. Hence, due to this advantage, the technic is relatively safe to the females during pregnancy and children especially, where the high radiation dose is very harmful. Moreover, the scanned images are of high-resolution giving sharper, faster, clearer and accurate images than x-ray film images. The digital images can immediately be stored in the computer memory for the future and permanent patient record. Thousands of such images can be stored this way and can be instantly recalled at any date in future. They can not only be easily retrieved but also can be combined and manipulated to supply more information. Hence, all the problems associated with x-ray films like storage and missing of x-rays can be eliminated. There is a definite improvement in diagnostic performance of this technic over the conventional radiography, in detecting hidden and not so easily seen carious lesions, apical pathology and pathologies of gums. Being ecofriendly in nature, the technique saves chemical waste associated with x-ray films and provides a great help in maintaining office hygiene as well.

INTRA-ORAL CAMERA

Intraoral camera is again a digital device and an integral part of the Innovative Digital Dentistry which has got built-in image capture facilities and provides the patient the finest imaging Intraoral photography. This is also an excellent Patient motivation and education device. Patient can view his or her dental condition while relaxing in a dental chair and also view the justification of required urgent or suggested treatment plan (by dentist) and very importantly the improvement or progress postoperatively.

BONE DENSITOMETER

Bone Densitometer is also an electronic device to measure bone density and very useful to find out the bone fracture risk in a patient. The device after examination gives the results within few seconds and is of great use in the patients undergoing Implant surgeries of teeth.

The Digital Dental Technology helps in every step of clinical procedure and save the time all through the procedure giving fast, accurate, long lasting treatment results by improving the prognosis of any specific case. With the advent of Digital imaging systems, the transmission of images to any part of the world has become possible through Internet to consult other specialists for diagnosis, conference or educational purposes. Although quite a handful of dental clinics are well equipped with such imaging systems, the Digital technology has no doubt come a long way and provides the best of services to mankind and very surely the technology of today and tomorrow.

Considering the numerous advantages obtained from the various computerized imaging technology the present and future dental patients can heave a sigh of relief for the cumbersome long hours can well be avoided at the dental clinics and not only quicker, but quality enhanced improved results would be gifted with.

CHAPTER 22
DENTAL IMPLANT – A REVOLUTION IN THE FIELD OF DENTISTRY

Dental Implant history dates back thousands of years and includes civilizations such as the ancient Chinese, who 4000 years ago inserted small bamboo sticks into the jawbone for fixed tooth replacement. The Egyptians and later physicians from Europe used ferrous and precious metals for implants over 2000 years ago, and the Incas used pieces of seashells, inserted into the jaw bones to replace missing teeth. The United States began its involvement in Implant Dentistry with Greenfield and his iridioplatinum cage in 1909. However, the latest Dental Implants, invented on the basis of scientific research, have been around in various forms since 1952.

Loosing teeth, either through old age or accident, is a cause of untold agony and depression for most of the patients. Even when elderly people start to lose their natural teeth and switch to dentures, the transition is not simple as they lose their sense of taste, resulting less intakes of food & subsequent weight loss, besides suffering discomfort such as nausea and vomiting. On the other hand, for the young, the loss of teeth causes an acute crisis of self-confidence. To give full satisfaction to the patient, with fixed restoration, artificial replacement of the roots of the teeth has always been the dream of the dental surgeon, which in turn led to the invention of Dental Implants. The technique of Dental Implantology promises a new quality of life to such persons having missing teeth, as it gives a person an opportunity to have an entirely new set of permanent teeth, fixed into the jawbone.

There are various anatomic and esthetic consequences of edentulism, which can be broadly grouped as follows:

(I) ANATOMIC PROBLEMS AND CONSEQUENCES ASSOCIATED WITH EDENTULISM

(1) Decreased width of supporting bone
(2) Decreased height of supporting bone
(3) Prominent mylohoid and internal oblique ridges
(4) Progressive decrease in Keratinized mucosa
(5) Prominent superior genial tubercles
(6) Elevation of prosthesis with contraction of mylohoid and buccinator muscles serving as

posterior support

(7) Forward movement of prosthesis from anatomic inclination

(8) Thinning of mucosa, with susceptibility to abrasion

(9) Loss of basal bone

(10) Paresthesia from dehiscent mandibular canal

(11) Increase in size of tongue

(12) More active role of tongue in mastication

(13) Decrease of neuromuscular control with aging

(14) Effect of bone loss on esthetic appearance of lower 1/3 of face

(II) ESTHETIC CONSEQUENCES OF EDENTULISM

(1) Prognathic appearance

(2) Decrease in horizontal labial angle

(3) Thinning of lips (especially of maxilla)

(4) Deepening of nasolabial groove

(5) Increased depth of associated vertical lines

(6) Decrease in facial height

(7) Loss of tone in muscles of facial expression

(8) Increased length of maxillary lip

(9) Less teeth shown at rest position and lower high lip-line position (aged smile)

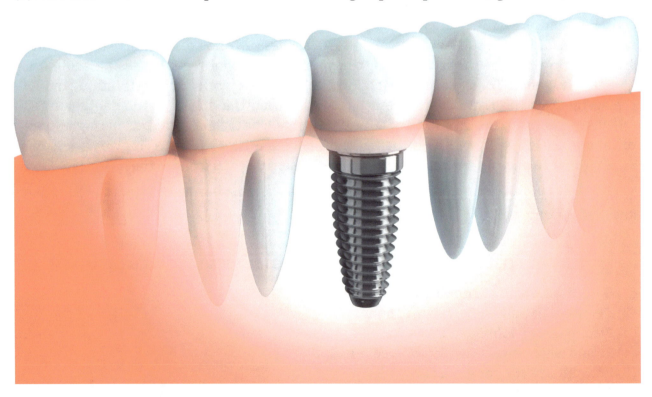

Dental Implant is the latest and most permanent tooth replacement option available today. The procedure of inserting of latest variety of Dental Implants is comparatively less cumbersome, painless with less postoperative discomfort to the patients. A Dental Implant, normally made out of Titanium or Vitallium alloy, is implanted into the jawbone by gently making a precise receptor site and left to heal for 3-6 months. During this phase bone heals fusing to implant, after which final replacement of tooth is placed on top of it. Generally, the entire surgical procedure is done under local anesthesia only.

There are many advantages of Implant supported prosthesis, for the restoration of one or more missing teeth. Some of the main advantages are as follows:

ADVANTAGES OF IMPLANT- SUPPORTED PROSTHESIS

(1) Maintenance of bone
(2) Maintenance of occlusal vertical dimension
(3) Tooth positioned for esthetics
(4) Proper occlusion
(5) Improved psychologic health
(6) Regained proprioception (occlusal awareness)
(7) Increased stability
(8) Improved phonetics
(9) Reduced removable prosthesis size (eliminating palate or flanges)
(10) Improved success rate of prosthesis
(11) Increases survival time of restoration
(12) Improved function of prosthesis
(13) Maintenance of muscles of mastication and facial expression

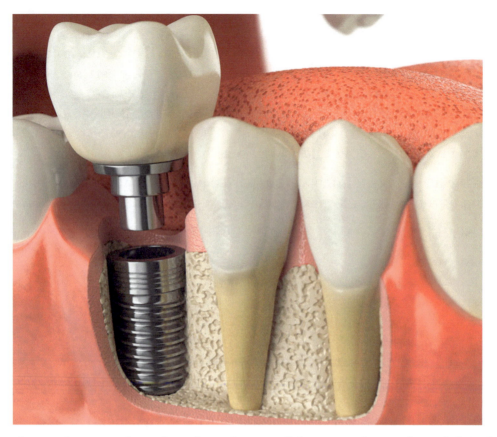

In modern times, the Dental Implantology is one of the most dynamic and fast developing specialization in the modern Dentistry. More than 100 types of major implant systems, promoted by different manufacturers, are available to the Dental Surgeons. Due to the availability of various types and forms of Implants, suitable in different conditions, the Dental Implants can be used in almost all the cases of partial or full edentulism. Like in the cases of the completely edentulism, where patient is having very thin ridge with loose dentures and where nothing much can be done, just 2 Micro Implants in each jaw can do wonders and give the unmatched and complete satisfaction to the patient, with Implant supported dentures. Even in the cases of Maxillary Sinus proximity or less Ridge height, the specialized Implants, which come in the size of as small as 5mm. length, can give excellent results. Even in the aesthetically important cases, dentist can put Immediate temporary bridge, by using Transitional Implants. In the cases where one has to go for extraction of one or more teeth, the dentist can insert the Screw Implants, in the socket immediately after the extraction, in the same sitting. So, with the latest advancement in the field of Dental Implantology, Dental Implants can be used in almost all the situations for replacement of one or more missing teeth. However, the Dental Surgeons know that the Dental implants are very technique sensitive and the dental implant may fail due to slight deviation of the accepted procedure.

Now most of the Dental Implant systems have the success rate of around 95%, if the operator observes proper surgical procedures. Apart from the overheating of the bone during preparation of receptor site in the jawbone which may cause early loss of Implant, improper load, angular load or improper sitting of prosthesis on dental implant, may create stress on a particular implant and may cause its failure in a long duration. So, all these factors should be observed during the treatment planning for a particular case, for the long-term success of this excellent technique of restoration of missing teeth. So, if the Dental Implants are placed with all the surgical skill, there are enough dental implants placed to support superstructure, superstructure placed on top of the dental implant is fabricated correctly, and the patient is not having any systemic or local contraindications for Implant surgery, then the chances are that these dental implants will be lasting foe patient's lifetime. However, patient need to keep oral hygiene and take care of the implant like the natural teeth.

Why are Implants preferred over Dentures and Bridges?

Dentures are generally loose and unstable. There are chances of falling out while talking and eating, and inability to pronounce properly, whereas implants can provide the stable dental replacements that is both functional and aesthetic.

Dentures and bridges require the grinding of adjacent healthy teeth on either side to support the bridge. When these teeth are lost at a later stage, the entire bridge needs replacement and grinding of the other teeth for new bridge. Implants are directly attached to the bone and gums, so no support of neighboring teeth is required as teeth are constructed over the Implants. Thus, neighboring teeth are spared of long-term problems.
Chewing efficiency of removable partial and complete dentures is only 20-25% of natural teeth, but for implanted teeth it can be 90-95%.

With Implants patient can enjoy better health through renewed eating habits. Implants also protect the jawbone from shrinkage and deterioration, which happen in case of bridge or Denture. Removable Dentures always give the artificial feeling of having some foreign body in the mouth, while Implant gives the natural feeling. With these invaluable benefits, the Implant treatment is becoming a fast-growing better alternative to the traditional tooth replacement methods.

CHAPTER 23
LASERS IN DENTISTRY

LASER

The term "LASER" is an abbreviation of: Light Amplification by Stimulated Emission of Radiation. Laser Technology was originated in 1960 and further advancements went on taking place since then. However, the history of soft laser therapy dates back 3000 to 4000 years ago. About 4000 years back, Egyptians were using photosensitization technic in the therapy of Vitiligo. They used a natural psoralen compound found in parsley, followed by exposure of the treated area to sunlight.

Over the last few years, Laser Therapy or more precisely LLLT (Low Level Laser Therapy) has become more widely used in the Medical, Dental and Veterinary practices. While the lasers like CO2 laser, ND: YAG, Argon etc. are labeled "High level lasers", others are "Low Level lasers". They are smaller, less expensive and work in milliwatts. The therapy performed with such lasers is called "Low Level Laser Therapy (LLLT)" or just "Laser therapy". They are also known as soft lasers or "therapeutic lasers". LLLT has been used as an alternative treatment modality where other therapies are insufficient or inadequate; there is a need to treat the patient sans drugs, may be as a patient's choice or in supplementary therapy, to relieve the pain quickly and to promote and shorten the postoperative healing period, as an adjunct to medication.

In the fields of Medicine and Surgery, the medical laser has been traditionally utilized to achieve photothermal destructive tissue reactions, with increased power densities. Nevertheless, reports are also suggestive of its therapeutic nonthermal effects. The most useful application of LLLT so far is in wound healing. Initially Laser was used for soft tissue lesions only but with the advancement, it has been possible to use it on hard tissues as well.

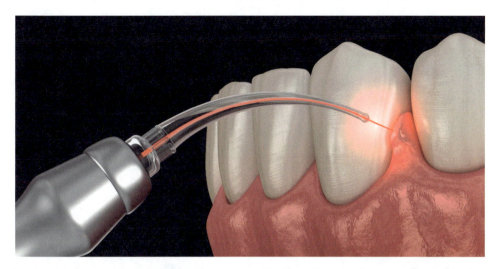

Laser is a device that produces high intensity light of a single wavelength, in such a fine parallel beam that it can be focused on to a very small spot. Unlike natural light which is composed of various electromagnetic fields traveling in disoriented fashion (incoherent), the light of a laser beam is coherent (waves all in same phase) and parallel. Hence, very high concentrations of energy can be achieved.

The name Laser has been derived from the lasing medium they contain, which provides them with power and particular wavelength. The basic elements in all the lasers are same, irrespective of their size, type or use. They need an active medium, which could be solid, liquid or gas; a source of energy, which is either electrical or high energy flash lamp and an optical resonator to stimulate and organize the photons into a narrow light beam. This light is then delivered to the target tissue by different mechanisms. The focused Laser beam in laser system usually applied to the surface of a lesion by the laser handpiece in each treatment session. Contact pressure laser therapy also sometimes tried in LLLT.

TYPES OF LASER

Laser can be either solid state (Ruby Laser, Nd: YAG Laser), Gas (Argon, CO_2 Laser) or of Excimer type (krypton Laser). Out of them Ruby, Nd: YAG, Argon and CO_2 Lasers are commonly used. The effect of laser therapy depends on the nature and chronicity of the disease. The clinical effect of laser therapy depends upon the amount of energy put into the tissues at each individual treatment point. In LLLT, treatment performed at such a low level that the temperature of the area to be treated would not exceed normal physiologic limits, i.e., around 36.5 C. The pulsed laser can penetrate tissues for several millimeters. The photochemical effects occur at level of the mitochondria. Laser stimulation can increase the Adenosine Triphosphate (ATP) levels in the cells and effect cellular functions. According to research, a treatment schedule of one daily exposure for 3-4 consecutive days enhances the effects of the laser treatment. Low energy irradiation affects the electrical activity (nerve conduction and active potentials) of an injured nerve. This effect lasts for at least 1 year following a short series of irradiation. There is minimum scar tissue development and enhancement of nerve tissue regeneration afterwards.

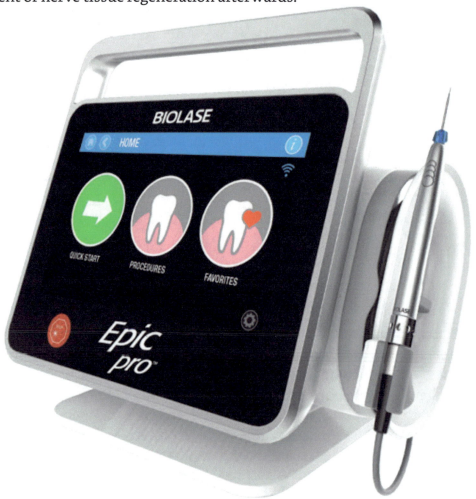

The analgesic effect of laser therapy is related to the duration of application, number of visits and reduction or elimination of pain. The findings of various clinicians in literature confirmed that satisfactory analgesic effects of laser treatment occurred after first or second session. In neuralgic disorders, patient receiving infrared laser therapy (A 904 nm low incident energy laser) receives immediate pain relief (by end of first treatment session). Long-term pain relief accounts for 1 year or more. Further pain reduction occurs with clinical improvement in the condition. Moreover, in the treatment of mouth ulcers and hypersensitivity of teeth, irradiation reduces or eliminates pain and promotes healing of ulcers without any side effects from laser irradiation.

Fundamental principles in LLLT Therapy-
(1) It should be performed with correct dosage
(2) It should be performed at the correct points (in acute diseases-around 5-10 mm and chronic disease around -10-15 mm)

(3) There should be correct distance between treatment points.

(4) There should be right interval between the treatments.

(5) It should be started as soon as possible after the problem arises.

Some Common Indications of Laser therapy in Dentistry

(1) Teeth extraction-Normal or Surgical

(2) All types of gums and periodontal surgeries

(3) Ulceration- minor or major Apthous ulcers

(4) Dental cavities management and treatment

(5) Endodontic (Root Canal Treatment) procedures

(6) Hypersensitivity in teeth

(7) Pain related to Nervous Origin Ex. Trigeminal Neuralgia, Facial Pain etc.

(8) Pain of muscular origin and traumatic disorders leading to Trismus or difficulty in opening mouth

(9) TMJ (Temporomandibular joint) disorders causing radiating pain in ENT region, discomfort and deformity

(10) Management of oral precancerous and cancerous lesions

Clinical effects of LLLT

(1) Pain relief- immediate and afterwards to postoperative

(2) Faster wound healing

(3) Minimum scar tissue formation

(4) Muscles relaxation leading to

(5) Reduction in discomfort, pain, anxiety

Structural or Biologic Effects of LLLT

(1) Cells regeneration

(2) Cellular growth stimulation

(3) Stimulating nerve function

(4) Reduction in fibrous tissue formation

(5) Anti-inflammatory effects

According to latest findings, quicker integration of implants, new bone formation and synthetic bone integration along with faster epithelialization by correct use of soft tissue laser treatment has indicated wide use of Laser therapy in implant surgeries as well.

With the gradual increase in standard of living and environmental factors favorable to life, world life expectancy has increased. Nevertheless, several nervous disorders and neuralgia such as Trigeminal neuralgia, migraine, post herpatic neuralgia, rheumatoid arthritis, low back pain, cervical spondylosis etc. are also showing steep rise due to present state of living of all of us. LLLT system has been found to be very effective in treatment of such conditions where other conventional therapies have been received with no or very little success.

The only major drawback has been with the laser technology is the high cost involved in the laser therapy compared to other conventional therapies. As such there is no side effect or adverse reaction has been observed in the laser therapy. Various useful applications of LLLT or laser therapy in Dentistry have been confirmed. Proper diagnosis, correct treatment planning and correct dosages in laser therapy are the factors of paramount importance in order to obtain better and satisfactory results. Last but not the least, while exploring the use of laser therapy for Dental decay causing various dental ailments, a breakthrough development in photodynamic therapy against bacteria eventually leads to a widespread use of lasers in Dentistry.

CHAPTER 24
PREVENTIVE AND COMMUNITY DENTISTRY

PREVENTIVE DENTISTRY

Preventive dentistry is a philosophy of dental practice dedicated to the prevention of dental diseases. It is neither a technique nor a series of procedures devoted to the prevention of dental diseases. The major objectives of preventive dentistry are: (1) to consider the patient in his or her entirety, (2) to maintain a healthy mouth in a state of optimal health as long as possible, (3) to prevent the initiation of oral disease, (4) to stop the progression of existing oral disease as soon as possible, (5) to provide the appropriate rehabilitation of form and function at the earliest possible time and as perfectly as possible, and (6) to provide the patient with the knowledge, skills, and motivations necessary to prevent the initiation, progression, and recurrence of dental disease.

PREVALENT DENTAL DISEASES AND ITS PREVENTION

Dental caries and periodontal disease are the most prevalent dental disease in modern society. About 98°% of the population is afflicted with dental caries. Though estimates vary, it is generally accepted that about 95% of the population suffers from one or another form of periodontal disease.

The two fundamental approaches for the prevention of dental caries are: (1) inhibition of the cariogenic factors attacking the tooth, namely, the cariogenic members(bacteria) of the oral flora, and (2) increasing the resistance of the tooth surface to acid demineralization.

The available measures for inhibiting the attacking forces are: (1) the removal of dental plaque by physical measures, namely, toothbrushing and flossing, and (2) reduction of the intake of fermentable carbohydrates, especially sucrose, and particularly the elimination of such foods between regular meals.

DENTAL PLAQUE

Dental plaque may be defined as a tenaciously adherent gelatinous mass comprised predominantly of bacterial colonies (70%) with the remainder consisting of water, food residues, desquamated epithelial cells, and white blood cells.

For the microorganisms to adhere to the tooth surfaces and colonize, bacterial enzymes (dextransucrases, levansucrases) degrade sucrose to form extracellular polysaccharides known as dextrans and levans. These latter polysaccharides facilitate the adhesion of the microorganisms to the pellicle-coated tooth surface. In the presence of food residues, the organisms then colonize forming dental plaque.

ROLE OF DIETARY FACTOR IN DENTAL CARIES

It is important to have a proper dietary analysis for dental purposes to check the cariogenic nature of the diet of an individual and society in general at community level. Dietary analysis is useful to measure the following factors:

1. Cariogenic potential of the diet.
2. Physical consistency of the diet.

The following factors determine the cariogenic potential of a dietary constituent:
1. Amount of sucrose (or readily fermentable carbohydrates) present in the food.
2. Amount of intraoral retention of food item (with particular consideration to the physical form of the food, i.e., liquid vs. solid, etc.).
3. Frequency of ingestion of the food (particularly if ingested between meals). It should be noted that, in general, the frequency of ingestion and the relative degree of intraoral retention are considered to have a greater impact on the cariogenic potential of a given food than the amount of sucrose present in that food.

The incidence of dental caries may be reduced as much as 50% through effective dietary counseling programs. Of particular importance in achieving such success is the elimination of highly retentive sucrose-containing foods and the use of nonsucrose-containing snack foods.

Some of the key factors for successful dietary counseling are:
1. Implement gradual changes one at a time, rather than drastic changes all at once.
2. Utilize dietary substitutions rather than outright elimination.
3. Utilize continual psychological reinforcement.

MULTIPLE FLUORIDE THERAPY

This term refers to the simultaneous use of several different types of fluoride treatments to provide the patient with the maximum degree of caries protection that may be achieved with fluorides. In practice this includes the ingestion of fluoride (i.e., communal fluoridation or fluoride tablets) during the period of tooth formation and maturation, posteruptive fluoride treatments (i.e., topical fluoride applications), and the daily home use of fluorides (i.e., dentifrices and mouth rinses).

COMMUNITY WATER FLUORIDATION

Community water fluoridation is the controlled adjustment of the fluoride content of the public water supply to an optimal concentration governed by the geographic location and climatic conditions for that community. Numerous clinical studies have shown that the ingestion of optimally fluoridated drinking water throughout the period of pre-eruptive tooth formation and posteruptive enamel maturation reduces the prevalence of dental caries 55% to 60%. This degree of caries protection is imparted to both the primary and permanent dentitions.

TOPICAL FLUORIDE APPLICATION

Topical fluoride application is the procedure of applying concentrated solutions of fluoride to the erupted dentition in the dental office for the prevention of dental caries.

The three systems for topical fluoride application that are recognized as being both safe and effective for the prevention of dental caries are (1) 2% sodium fluoride solution, (2) 8% stannous fluoride solution, and (3) acidulated phosphate fluoride (APF) solutions or gels having a fluoride concentration of 1.23% with a pH of about 3.5.

The topical application of concentrated solutions of fluoride to the teeth results in the formation of chemical reaction products on the enamel surface that make the tooth surface more resistant to enamel demineralization. The use of topical fluoride applications should be considered for any patient with active caries and as a preventive measure for children particularly during the period when the development of caries is more probable (i.e., up to 15 years of age). Multiple fluoride treatments may be expected to arrest incipient carious lesions as well as prevent new caries formation. Thus, such treatments are particularly useful for children, and, while all three approved systems are beneficial, the treatments of choice are stannous fluoride and acidulated phosphate fluoride. In adults, only stannous fluoride has been shown to be of significant value. The frequency for reapplication should be dictated by the caries activity of the patient. With active caries, fluoride treatments should be given at least each 3 to 6 months whereas annual treatments may be adequate as a preventive measure.

PUBLIC DENTAL HEALTH

Public Health is the science and art of:

a)   Preventing disease

b)   Prolonging life

c)   Promoting health and efficiency through organized community effort.

Winslow (1920) stated that "the benefit of organized health is to enable every citizen to realize the birth right of health and longevity.

Public Health is precisely, to plan and organize the channels of, health, in accordance with the geographic, demographic, social and cultural conditions of the country for the welfare of common man in rural or urban areas.

Dental Public health is the art and science of:

a)   Preventing the incidence of dental diseases

b)   Prolonging the life span of dentition.

c)   Promoting dental health and efficiency through organized community efforts.

d)   Providing to adopt methods to check up the disease.

e)   Providing statistical data and research opportunities.

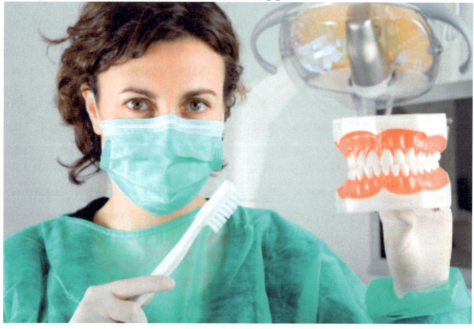

RESPONSIBILITY OF PUBLIC HEALTH DENTIST IN BASIC HEALTH UNIT FOR

DENTAL CARE

The dental professionals working at community level should follow the following responsibilities:

(1) To apply known preventive measures for the control of the disease from the community.

(2) To diagnose the disease for treatment or reference to specialist.

(3) To understand the contribution of dental science, its development, research and service.

(4) To understand and have the idea of basic knowledge, evaluate its development and techniques of application of technical knowledge to the existing dental problems.

(5) To recognize its responsibility towards patients and community as community workers.

(6) To adopt the new situation-emergency and develop a judgment to decide the case on the spot.

(7) To have the ability for planning a care program and methodology for improvement of the existing system.

(8) To identify all aspects of oral health problems and to assist in planning, implementation, and evaluation of oral health.

CHAPTER 25
DENTAL ETHICS

Dentistry, like medicine, is a Hippocratic profession. It has developed and now uses a set of techniques that have evolved rapidly and discernibly within the few decades. Hippocrates incorporated into his school of thoughts three ingredients which have survived into contemporary health care practice:

First, there was a skill or art which was learned by apprenticeship in dealing with actual cases.
Second, there was a search for the natural explanations of disease and an attempt to build up a body of scientific knowledge which could be used to inform one's skill.
Third, there was an ethos of caring and respect for human beings.

The first two elements made the Hippocratic approach to medicine a suitable foundation for a tradition of health care apt to continue into a scientific age. The third element of the Hippocratic approach is the one most often remembered because it has survived in the Hippocratic Oath. It guards medical practice against the unscrupulous use of that specialized and privileged knowledge which has been obtained in an attempt to offer real benefits to suffering people. The Hippocratic school was so concerned that the art they practiced should be surrounded by the ethical commitments which they considered important that their oath included the words:
I will impart a knowledge of the Art to my own sons and those of my teachers and to the disciples bound by a stipulation and oath according to the law of medicine but to no other.

The implication of this underlying ethical commitment is that any Hippocratic professional must primarily share a caring ethos and that only on that basis was he fit to learn the specialized skills of clinical care. The Hippocratic stress on caring and benefit is often misinterpreted as expressing a relative neglect, in health care practice, of the respect for the patient as a person.

The value commitments of the Hippocratic tradition can, however, create conflicts in practice-for instance, between the desire for standardized and comprehensive knowledge and the need to respect persons as individuals. Despite these conflicts, such commitments remain an inescapable part of the proper function of a health care profession. Therefore, we must find ethical resolutions to the various conflicts that can arise if we are to practice properly as Hippocratic professionals.

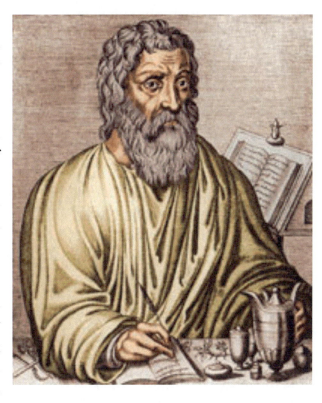

The dental profession holds a special position of trust within society. Consequently, society affords the profession certain privileges that are not available to members of the public-at-large. In return, the profession is supposed to make a commitment to society that its members will adhere to high ethical standards of conduct. It has always been expected that the dentists follow high ethical standards which have the benefit of the patient as their primary goal. In recognition of this goal, the education and training of a dentist has resulted in society affording to the profession the privilege and obligation of self-government. To fulfill this privilege, the high ethical standards should be adopted and practiced throughout the dental school educational process and subsequent professional career.

To come true to the professional expectations in the society, the dentists should possess not only knowledge, skill, and technical competence but also those traits of character that foster adherence to ethical principles. Qualities of honesty, compassion, kindness, integrity, fairness, and charity are part of the ethical education of a dentist and practice of dentistry and help to define the true professional. As such, each dentist should share in providing advocacy to and care of the underserved. It is urged that the dentist meet this goal, subject to individual circumstances, and the ethical dentist should strive to do that which is right and good.

The American Dental Association has documented the expected principals of ethics and professional conduct on the part of the dental professionals, the collection of which is known as ADA Code. Members of the ADA voluntarily agree to abide by the ADA Code as a condition of membership in the Association. They recognize that continued public trust in the dental profession is based on the commitment of individual dentists to high ethical standards of conduct.

The ADA Code has three main components: The Principles of Ethics, the Code of Professional Conduct and the Advisory Opinions.

The Principles of Ethics are the aspirational goals of the profession. They provide guidance and offer justification for the Code of Professional Conduct and the Advisory Opinions. There are five fundamental principles that form the foundation of the ADA Code: patient autonomy, nonmaleficence (do no harm), beneficence, justice and veracity. The Code of Professional Conduct is an expression of specific types of conduct that are either required or prohibited.

Although ethics and the law are closely related, they are not the same. Ethical obligations may, and often do, exceed the legal duties. In resolving any ethical problem, dentists should consider the ethical principles, the patient's needs and interests, and any applicable laws.

IMPORTANT PRINCIPALS OF DENTAL ETHICS

1. **Self Determination:** The dentist has a duty to respect the patient's rights to self-determination and confidentiality.

This principle expresses the concept that professionals have a duty to treat the patient according to the patient's desires, within the bounds of accepted treatment, and to protect the patient's confidentiality. Under this principle, the dentist's primary obligations include involving patients in treatment decisions in a meaningful way, with due consideration being given to the patient's needs, desires, and abilities, and safeguarding the patient's privacy.

2. **Patient Involvement:** The dentist should inform the patient of the proposed treatment, and any reasonable alternatives, in a manner that allows the patient to become involved in treatment decisions.

3. **Patient Records:** Dentists are obliged to safeguard the confidentiality of patient records. Dentists shall maintain patient records in a manner consistent with the protection of the welfare of the patient. Upon request of a patient or another dental practitioner, dentists shall provide any information in accordance with applicable law that will be beneficial for the future treatment of that patient.

4. **Furnishing Copies of Records:** A dentist has the ethical obligation on request of either the patient or the patient's new dentist to furnish in accordance with applicable law, either

gratuitously or for nominal cost, such dental records or copies or summaries of them, including dental X-rays or copies of them, as will be beneficial for the future treatment of that patient. This obligation exists whether or not the patient's account is paid in full.

5. Nonmaleficence (do no harm): The dentist has a duty to refrain from harming the patient.

This principle expresses the concept that professionals have a duty to protect the patient from harm. Under this principle, the dentist's primary obligations include keeping knowledge and skills current, knowing one's own limitations and when to refer to a specialist or other professional, and knowing when and under what circumstances delegation of patient care to auxiliaries is appropriate.

6. Education: The privilege of dentists to be accorded professional status rests primarily in the knowledge, skill, and experience with which they serve their patients and society. All dentists, therefore, have the obligation of keeping their knowledge and skill current.

7. Consultation and Referral: Dentists shall be obliged to seek consultation, if possible, whenever the welfare of patients will be safeguarded or advanced by utilizing those who have special skills, knowledge, and experience. When patients visit or are referred to specialists or consulting dentists for consultation:

1. The specialists or consulting dentists upon completion of their care shall return the patient, unless the patient expressly reveals a different preference, to the referring dentist, or, if none, to the dentist of record for future care.

2. The specialists shall be obliged when there is no referring dentist and upon a completion of their treatment to inform patients when there is a need for further dental care.

8. Second Opinions: A dentist who has a patient referred by a third party for a "second opinion" regarding a diagnosis or treatment plan recommended by the patient's treating dentist should render the requested second opinion in accordance with this Code of Ethics. In the interest of the patient being afforded quality care, the dentist rendering the second opinion should not have a vested interest in the ensuing recommendation.

9. Use of Auxiliary Personnel: Dentists shall be obliged to protect the health of their patients by only assigning to qualified auxiliaries those duties which can be legally delegated. Dentists shall be further obliged to prescribe and supervise the patient care provided by all auxiliary personnel working under their direction.

10. Personal Impairment: It is unethical for a dentist to practice while abusing controlled substances, alcohol or other chemical agents which impair the ability to practice. All dentists have an ethical obligation to urge chemically impaired colleagues to seek treatment. Dentists with first-hand knowledge that a colleague is practicing dentistry when so impaired have an ethical responsibility to report such evidence to the professional ethical and legal bodies of dental council.

11. Ability to Practice: A dentist who contracts any disease or becomes impaired in any way that might endanger patients or dental staff shall, with consultation and advice from a qualified physician or other authority, limit the activities of practice to those areas that do not endanger patients or dental staff.

12. Postexposure, Bloodborne Pathogens: All dentists, regardless of their bloodborne pathogen status, have an ethical obligation to immediately inform any patient who may have been exposed to blood or other potentially infectious material in the dental office of the need for post exposure evaluation and follow-up and to immediately refer the patient to a qualified health care practitioner who can provide postexposure services. The dentist's ethical obligation in the event of an exposure incident extends to providing information concerning the dentist's own bloodborne pathogen status to the evaluating health care practitioner, if the dentist is the source individual, and to submitting to testing that will assist in the evaluation of the patient. If a staff member or other third person is the source individual, the dentist should encourage that person to cooperate as needed for the patient's evaluation.

13. Patient Abandonment: Once a dentist has undertaken a course of treatment, the dentist should not discontinue that treatment without giving the patient adequate notice and the opportunity to obtain the services of another dentist. Care should be taken that the patient's oral health is not jeopardized in the process.

14. Personal Relationships with Patients: Dentists should avoid interpersonal relationships that could impair their professional judgment or risk the possibility of exploiting the confidence placed in them by a patient.

15. Community Service: Since dentists have an obligation to use their skills, knowledge and experience for the improvement of the dental health of the public and are encouraged to be leaders in their community, dentists in such service shall conduct themselves in such a manner as to maintain or elevate the esteem of the profession.

16. Research and Development: Dentists have the obligation of making the results and benefits of their investigative efforts available to all when they are useful in safeguarding or promoting the health of the public.

17. Patient Selection: While dentists, in serving the public, may exercise reasonable discretion in selecting patients for their practices, dentists shall not refuse to accept patients into their practice or deny dental service to patients because of the patient's race, creed, color, sex or national origin.

18. Patients with bloodborne pathogens: A dentist has the general obligation to provide care to those in need. A decision not to provide treatment to an individual because the individual is infected with Human Immunodeficiency Virus, Hepatitis B Virus, Hepatitis C Virus or another bloodborne pathogen, based solely on that fact, is unethical. Decisions with regard to the type of dental treatment provided or referrals made or suggested should be made on the same basis as they are made with other patients. As is the case with all patients, the individual dentist should determine if he or she has the need of another's skills, knowledge, equipment, or experience. The dentist should also determine, after consultation with the patient's physician, if appropriate, if the patient's health status would be significantly compromised by the provision of dental treatment.

19. Emergency Service: Dentists shall be obliged to make reasonable arrangements for the emergency care of their patients of record. Dentists shall be obliged when consulted in an emergency by patients not of record to make reasonable arrangements for emergency care. If treatment is provided, the dentist, upon completion of treatment, is obliged to return the patient to his or her regular dentist unless the patient expressly reveals a different preference.

20. Overbilling: It is unethical for a dentist to increase a fee to a patient solely because the patient is covered under a dental benefits plan.

21. Unnecessary Services: A dentist who recommends and performs unnecessary dental services or procedures is engaged in unethical conduct.

22. Marketing or Sale of products or procedures: Dentists who, in the regular conduct of their practices, engage in or employ auxiliaries in the marketing or sale of products or procedures to their patients must take care not to exploit the trust inherent in the dentist-patient relationship for their own financial gain. Dentists should not induce their patients to purchase products or undergo procedures by misrepresenting the product's value, the necessity of the procedure or the dentist's professional expertise in recommending the product or procedure.

22. Professional Announcement: In order to properly serve the public, dentists should represent themselves in a manner that contributes to the esteem of the profession. Dentists should not misrepresent their training and competence in any way that would be false or misleading in any material respect.

23. Advertising: No dentist shall advertise or solicit patients in any form of communication in a manner that is false or misleading in any material respect.

24. Unearned, Non-health degrees: A dentist may use the title Doctor or Dentist, DDS, MS or any additional earned, advanced academic degrees in health service areas in an announcement to the public. The announcement of an unearned academic degree may be misleading because of the likelihood that it will indicate to the public the attainment of specialty or diplomate status. An unearned academic degree is one which is awarded by an educational institution not accredited by a generally recognized accrediting body or is an honorary degree. The use of a non-health degree in an announcement to the public may be a representation which is misleading because the public is likely to assume that any degree announced is related to the qualifications of the dentist as a practitioner. Some organizations grant dentists fellowship status as a token of membership in the organization or some other form of voluntary association. The use of such fellowships in advertising to the general public may be misleading because of the likelihood that it will indicate to the public attainment of education or skill in the field of dentistry. Generally, unearned, or non-health degrees and fellowships that designate association, rather than attainment, should be limited to scientific papers and curriculum vitae. In all instances, state law should be consulted. In any review by the dental council of the use of designations in advertising to the public, the council will apply the standard of whether the use of such is false or misleading in a material respect.

25. Name of Practice: Since the name under which a dentist conducts his or her practice may be a factor in the selection process of the patient, the use of a trade name or an assumed name that is false or misleading in any material respect is unethical. Use of the name of a dentist no longer actively associated with the practice may be continued for a period not to exceed one year.

26. Credentials in General Dentistry: General dentists may announce fellowships or other credentials earned in the area of general dentistry so long as they avoid any communications that express or imply specialization and the announcement includes the disclaimer that the dentist is a general dentist. The use of abbreviations to designate credentials shall be avoided when such use would lead the reasonable person to believe that the designation represents an academic degree, when such is not the case.

NEEDS FOR THE FUTURE

Ethical and legal dilemmas and violations occur daily in the practice of dentistry. Occurrences of gross violations often surprise and appall those who conscientiously adhere to the profession's ethical standards. While the association between ethics and patient care is an obvious and important one, ethical sensitivity and behavior are also necessary before students begin their clinical experiences. The authors feel that the dental ethics courses should be offered, not as electives, but as a regular subject at the dental professional schools, as it is of paramount importance, particularly in the present situation when "most of the sources that transmit moral standards have declined in importance" or seem to have declined in the minds of most people. Dental training programs are required to teach ethics and are charged with producing graduates who are "competent in the application of the principles of ethical reasoning and professional responsibility as they pertain to patient care and practice management.

Continuing Education

Regardless of the student's level of mastery of ethics knowledge, continuing education is critical to maintain competency and ensure lifelong learning. The history of dental ethics education demonstrates the profession's commitment to promoting the ethical behavior of dentists. Significant strides in both content and approach over the last quarter century indicate that, in many dental schools in Canada, ethics is being taught early and often and in a format that emphasizes self-reflection and moral reasoning, making it important a thorough revamping of the curriculum of the subject of Dental Ethics.

CHAPTER 26
COMMON DISEASES ENCOUNTERED IN THE DENTAL OFFICE

The health professional working in a dental office is exposed to many diseases on a daily basis including the herpes viruses and possibly hepatitis B, AIDS, and tuberculosis. Some of the serious diseases the operator may encounter in the dental office quite often, are discussed below.

Herpes Viruses

The word "herpes" comes from the ancient Greek word Herpein (to creep) the Greeks believed that herpes sores crept over the body. There are as many as 50 different types of herpes viruses that may attack the animal kingdom. The five types of herpes viruses that occur in humans are:

· Herpes simplex virus type 1
· Herpes simplex virus type 2
· Varicella-zoster virus
· Epstein-Barr virus
· Cytomegalovirus.

Because these viruses belong to the same family, they share common physical characteristics— size, shape, structure, and internal composition.

Herpes Simplex

The diseases classified as herpes simplex are systemic viral infections. They are characterized by:

1. A localized primary lesion,
2. Latency (the virus can remain hidden in the body),
3. The tendency of the virus to recur periodically.

The herpes simplex virus can be found anywhere in the body and it attacks all segments of the population. Once a person has been infected with a herpes virus, it will remain with the human body for the rest of the life, although recurring infections diminish in intensity and duration. Herpes simplex type 1 and type 2 are separate and distinct infections. Herpes simplex virus type 1 is usually found above the waist— most often on the face, mouth, or lips in the form of fever blisters, cold sores, or canker sores. The incubation period is between 2 and 12 days, and the virus is highly contagious. The patient will have fever initially accompanied by enlarged cervical lymph nodes, malaise, and burning or pruritus (itching) in the areas of the lesions. Infection is caused by direct contact with the saliva of infected persons, by touching active cold sores, and by kissing persons who have fever blisters on their lips or face. Herpes simplex type 2 usually settles below the waist in the genital area. The virus may also produce sores on the anus, buttocks, or inner thighs. Genital herpes is the most common sexually transmitted disease in the North America. Herpes simplex virus type 2 is transmitted through direct contact with saliva, or secretions from mucous membranes and lesions of infected persons and may be transmitted sexually.

Varicella-Zoster Virus

The herpes virus varicella-zoster is responsible for chicken pox (varicella) in young people and shingles (herpes zoster) in adults. Varicella virus is extremely communicable before the rash appears and until the sores have crusted over. The virus enters the body through the respiratory mucous membranes and causes systemic disease characterized by high fever, malaise, and skin lesions, which may appear anywhere on the body.

Epstein-Barr Virus

Epstein-Barr virus is another of the herpes viruses. It causes mononucleosis, commonly known as "mono." Since the virus is transmitted in saliva by prolonged direct contact, probably through kissing, it is also called the "kissing disease." The disease occurs mostly in adolescents and young adults. It is characterized by high fever, inflammation of the pharynx (sore throat), and swelling of the lymph glands. Treatment involves bed rest and good diet over a long period of time.

Cytomegalovirus

Cytomegalovirus (CMV) is another member of the herpes virus group. This virus is quite common and usually does not produce symptoms. It is similar to herpes type 1 and type 2 in that it remains hidden in body tissues and has the ability to produce recurrent infections just as herpes simplex types 1 and 2 do. CMV is dangerous to pregnant women because it also crosses into the placenta and can produce very serious congenital infections in the fetus. CMV can be found in all body secretions including saliva, blood, urine, semen, cervical secretions, and breast milk. Transmitting CMV from one person to another requires prolonged direct contact with secretions and excretions. When there are symptoms at all, they are like those of mononucleosis.

Hepatitis B

Hepatitis, an infectious inflammation of the liver, is the third most communicable disease in North America. The virus is transmitted more easily than HIV and is a greater threat than most people realize. Hepatitis infections can be mild or severe. Most people recover from hepatitis without any complications. Some people, however, develop chronic forms of this disease. The period of time between contact with the virus and appearance in the blood can be as short as two weeks, but usually averages 60 to 90 days. Symptoms may appear from four weeks to six months after exposure. Ninety percent of otherwise healthy adults with hepatitis B will recover completely. The virus is transmitted or spread by direct contact with bodily secretions of people who are ill with the disease or who have a chronic infection. If a pregnant woman has the disease, her infant may get the virus through contact with her blood at birth. The virus can live on countertops or other surfaces for several days. OSHA regulations must be strictly followed concerning handpiece spray, needle stick, or puncture from contaminated instruments. The dental staff should be immunized against hepatitis and must take necessary steps to protect herself or himself from this disease. Hepatitis B can be prevented by immunization. The Academy of Pediatrics now recommends that all newborns be immunized against serum hepatitis (HBV). Two vaccines are available for use against hepatitis B virus. Three injections given intramuscularly in the deltoid muscle of the arm for adults and in the thigh for infants and young children are required to immunize against hepatitis. The second vaccination should be given one month after the first, and the third vaccination should be given six months after the first. The dental staff is exposed to this disease by patients who are carriers (the virus remains in the body for life). Since the risk of hepatitis is one of the occupational risks for the dental team, one need to be aware of the pathology of the disease and adequate protection is very important. In addition to immunization there are other precautions and protective measures which one need to follow in day-to-day practice.

AIDS

"AIDS" is a word formed from the phrase acquired immunodeficiency syndrome. Human immunodeficiency virus (HIV) is the virus that causes the collection of symptoms known as AIDS. HIV infection begins a long, slow process that leads to the destruction of the body's immune system, the system that keeps the body free from disease. There are five phases or stages of development of HIV infection. The virus may be transmitted during any phase or stage of infection. The first phase lasts from four weeks to six months, during which time the virus will not show up in the blood. The second phase is characterized by a short period of flulike symptoms, which include fever, skin rash, malaise, and swollen glands, and is called the acute primary HIV infection stage. The third period may last from a year to 15 or 20 years, depending upon how healthy the infected person's immune system was at the time of infection, and how well he/she has taken care of them. Even though there are no symptoms, the disease can be detected through laboratory tests. This third phase is called asymptomatic HIV infection. When the infected person starts to have symptoms indicating the immune system is beginning to be suppressed, the fourth phase has begun. These symptoms may include low grade fever, night sweats, diarrhea, unintended weight loss, swollen glands, sores in the mouth, and fatigue, among others. When any of these symptoms are present, the disease is approaching the stage when AIDS will be diagnosed. This usually occurs in about two or three years. AIDS is now diagnosed in this fifth phase. The Centers for Disease Control (CDC) sets guidelines to make sure that physicians reporting AIDS cases are using the same standards to diagnose patients. The CDC lists the conditions, which must be present for a diagnosis of AIDS. Once AIDS is finally diagnosed, 80 to 90 percent of the patients die within three years.

Transmission of HIV

HIV can be transmitted in several ways. It is transmitted from person to person through sexual relations. An infected mother may pass the virus through the placenta to her baby and through breast-feeding. It may be transmitted indirectly by contaminated blood transfusions, by using contaminated needles, or by direct contact with infected blood or body fluids on mucous membranes or open wounds. The Dental Staff must protect themselves from possible infection by considering each patient to be a potential transmitter of the virus. They must use the required protective clothing and other measures to ensure themselves and others as much protection from transmission or contraction of the virus as possible.

Oral Manifestations of AIDS

The oral cavity is one of the first areas of the body to show possible symptoms of AIDS. The most common fungal infection seen in AIDS patients is due to a yeast called Candida Albicans (thrush). Thrush is a persistent, creamy white, curd-like patch that coats the tongue, throat, and esophagus. It causes pain and may lead to difficulty in chewing and swallowing. Another condition similar to thrush is hairy leukoplakia, often seen in AIDS patients. Grayish-white lesions or patchy discolorations on the sides of or beneath the tongue that cannot be rubbed off are characteristic of this disease. Kaposi's sarcoma is another disease that is common in dental patients having AIDS. Small, red or purple lesions begin the disease, which then progresses for several years. Kaposi's sarcoma was seldom life threatening until the AIDS outbreak. When AIDS patients are relatively young, the Kaposi's sarcoma that affects them is very aggressive and progresses rapidly. The Kaposi's sarcoma that affects AIDS patients produces purplish, raised lesions on the mucous lining of the mouth, the trunk, the lymph nodes, and various internal organs. The first lesions often appear on the face and head and in the oral cavity. Unfortunately, Kaposi's sarcoma is fatal among HIV infected persons. As mentioned earlier, herpes simplex virus types 1 (HSV-1) and 2 (HSV-2) have the ability to remain latent in the body tissues and to become reactivated periodically. Herpes simplex type 2 is extremely common in AIDS patients. Since the immune system in AIDS patients does not function as well as in healthy people, the herpes simplex virus recurs more frequently in AIDS patients. The herpes simplex virus is associated with two types of cancer often seen in AIDS patients: cancer of the tongue with

HSV-1 and cancer of the rectum with HSV-2.

Tuberculosis and Other Lung Disorders

For many years, tuberculosis (TB) was not common in most of the developed countries. However, this highly contagious disease is coming back. In the past, patients were treated in isolation (in sanitariums) for 9 to 18 months. Medication was discovered to cure it, although many patients neglected to take it properly. Now there is a drug-resistant strains that is breaking out in hospitals and prisons—institutions where there are large numbers of people living in limited space. Patients who have the disease need no special dental treatment precautions. However, the dental team must take appropriate precautions. Patients with other lung diseases (emphysema, asthma, etc.) may experience difficulty breathing during procedures. Therefore, the operator must pay attention to any signs of discomfort or changes in respiration in these patients.

CHAPTER 27
DENTAL RECORDS AND DENTISTRY

A dental record is the detailed document of the history of the illness, physical examination, diagnosis, treatment, and management of a patient. Dental records are produced during a dental examination and are the recording of the state of a patient's teeth. The dental profession has an ethical and legal responsibility for patient care. Dental professionals are compelled by law to produce and maintain adequate patient records. A properly maintained patient record is a very important aspect of the patient care. In general, a "record" can be defined as information generated in the course of an organisation's official transactions and one that is documented to act as a source of reference and a tool by which an organisation is governed.

Dental Records Management

Dental records are essential for dentist and patient protection, and its maintenance is considered an ethical and legal obligation of the dentist: Ethical, because it satisfies the duty of care that the dentist has toward his patient and legal, as it is an investment for future protection against medico-legal complications. Comprehensive and accurate records are a vital part of dental practice. The primary purpose of maintaining dental records is to deliver quality patient care and follow-up. Dental records can also be used for forensic purposes and have an important role in teaching and research, as well as in legal matters.

Dental records and charts are permanent legal documents. They must be accurate and complete. A forensic pathologist, for example, may need to rely on dental records to identify a victim or missing person. Professional, ethical and legal responsibilities dictate that a record documenting all aspects of a patient's dental care be maintained. All patient records must be well organized, legible, readily accessible and understandable.

Electronic Records (EDR) and Record-keeping

Electronic Dental Records (EDR) must be able to visually display and print the recorded clinical and financial information for each client in chronological order and can print this information without unreasonable delay. They need to Include a password or otherwise provides reasonable protection against unauthorized access and back up files on a removable media and allows for data recovery or provides by other means reasonable protection against loss, damage, and/or inaccessibility of client information. EDR must be able to store the original data in a read-only format from within the dental program itself but protects the data files from entry and alteration from the database.

The use of electronic recordkeeping, including digital radiography is quite common. However, it is important to note that electronic records must comply with the requirements and regulations as established by the governing body such as the Royal College of Dental Surgeons, College of Dental Hygienists, etc.

Important points related to EDR
- The most important aspect of recordkeeping is accuracy of the record and safety in storage.
- The EDRs must have a login and password to access the data, or otherwise provide reasonable protection against unauthorized access, and can authenticate all entries
- EDRs must protect the original content of the recorded information when changed or updated
- EDRs need to record the date of each entry for each client in respect to the financial or clinical record and is capable of being printed separately from the recorded information for each client
- They need to provide access to the clinical and financial records of every client by their names
- They need to make easy to print or transfer all the original and modified entries.

Uses of Dental Records-Paper/Electronic Form
A properly maintained dental record has several uses as follows:
- Dental records are recordings from initial entry of patient information to assessing expertise of the dental professional to diagnose, treat, use resources and practice evidence-based dentistry.
- Dental records enable monitoring of the patients' state of oral health and can also be used to aid motivation in preventive oral healthcare practices.
- Clinical records are essential for delivery of good dental care, for ensuring continuity and completeness of dental treatment.
- A complete record also enables communication with another practitioner for communication and consultation purposes.
- It is helpful in monitoring the success/failure of any treatment carried out.
- A detailed and accurate dental record is essential as it serves the dentists own best interests in the event of a malpractice suit.
- Dental records are essential for dental audit, which is a vital part of quality control.
- Dental records can play a crucial role in forensic dentistry in identification, detection and solution of a crime, in civil proceedings or in natural or manmade disaster situations.
- Records can be used in the management and planning of health care facilities and

services, for health care research and the production of health care statistics.
•   Dental records reflect the quality of life as assessed by the patient and the dental professional.

Maintenance of accurate recordkeeping
•   All client charts must be in accordance with the standards of practice guidelines provided by the provincial governing body
•   All client charts must contain signed patient consent for treatment
•   All client charts must contain a currently updated and complete medical history
•   All charting entries must be recorded in the computer system or by hand in permanent ink
•   All entries in the dental chart must be signed, initialed or otherwise attributable to the attending provider
•   An explanation of the overall treatment plan, treatment alternatives, any risks or limitations of treatment and the estimated costs of the treatment must be provided to every client, parent or guardian or appropriate representative.
•   Radiographs and diagnostic aids must be properly labeled and dated.

Confidentiality, privacy, and protection of dental records and EDRs
Confidentiality is crucial to the relationship and trust between you and your patients. All patients' information acquired by any member of the dental team in their professional capacity is confidential. It should be protected from unauthorised disclosure in any condition. Client signed consent must be obtained prior to the release of any information requested from another dentist, the client's physician or authorized representative. Moreover, the confidentiality of records-paper or EDR must be respected and protected at all times. A record of oral or written communication with the client's primary care physician must be retained as part of the permanent record. It is important to store identical data in different places on several hard disks to improve system performance and data protection. It is advisable to use network management software to notify you through pagers and/or e-mail if potential hardware or software problems are detected and use Windows updates or automatic updates to protect your operating system. Regular disk cleanup utility to remove unnecessary files and free up hard drive space is essential.

Although the extent of detail required for each individual dental record must vary from client to client, certain baseline data must be included in accordance with guidelines as set out by the regulatory body. Document procedures to help recover your system and review, update and test of recovery procedures are important.

Important points about Personal Health Information (PHI)
PHI stands for Protected Health Information and is any information in a medical/dental record that can be used to identify an individual, and that was created, used, or disclosed in

the course of providing a health care service, such as a diagnosis or treatment.

PHI is a plan or service Relates to the payments or eligibility for health care in respect to the individual.

PHI relates to his/her physical or mental health

PHI Relates to providing health care, including identifying a provider of health care

PHI Can be a health number

Is in a record that contains any of the above information

Ontario's Personal Health Information Protection Act, 2004 (PHIPA), establishes rules for the collection, use and disclosure of personal health information by dentists and other health information custodians practicing in Ontario. The Information and Privacy Commissioner of Ontario created a useful Frequently Asked Questions guide on PHIPA and associated regulations in September 2015. While dentists should maintain current knowledge of their obligations under PHIPA, including reading articles published by the College and seeking legal advice as required, this FAQ can help dentists understand the Act and how it applies to them as well as provide information about individuals' rights with respect to their personal health information, which may interest patients and their parents, guardians or substitute decision-makers.

DENTAL RECORDKEEPING
Retention of PHI and Dental Records
The Guidelines of the Royal College of Dental Surgeons of Ontario contain practice parameters and standards that should be considered by all Ontario dentists in the care of their patients. These Guidelines may be used by the College or other bodies to determine if appropriate standards of practice and professional responsibilities have been maintained. Dentists are legally required to keep dental records. Clinical and financial patient records, as well as radiographs, consultant reports, and drug and lab prescriptions must be maintained for at least ten years after the date of the last entry in the patient's record. The same retention period applies to appointment books and other office records (such as equipment maintenance records, sterilization log and drug register).

Dentists have professional, legal, and ethical responsibilities to maintain a complete record of each patient's dental care. Clear, accurate and up-to-date patient records are essential to the delivery of high-quality care. Patient records must be well-organized, legible, understandable, and readily accessible. They remind the dentist of past and present conditions of the patient and treatments already provided, and they facilitate communication with other practitioners involved in the patient's care. For effective continuity of care, another dentist should be able to review the record easily and carry on with the patient's treatment.

Retention of dental records is minimum of 10 years. There are two exceptions-
  1. Working models do not have to be retained, however, diagnostic and statistical manuals

as a part of the permanent patient record should be kept for 10 years.

2. Copies of dental claims must be maintained for two years from the date of claim. An electronic copy of claims on a properly backed up system would be acceptable.

In the case of a minor, these records must be kept for at least ten years from the date the patient turned 18 years of age. Copies of dental claim forms must be kept for at least two years from the date the claim was provided to the patient or submitted on the patient's behalf.

Privacy Policy and Procedures

Client charts are considered part of the confidential record and shall be handled and processed accordingly. It is the responsibility of the health care provider to protect the personal health information contained in the charts while treating patients and exercising sensitivity to privacy. If a client has questions or concerns about the privacy of their information, they shall be directed to the Privacy Officer.

Personal Health Information Protection Act (PHIPA) and Dentistry

The Personal Health Information Protection Act relates to the delivery of health care to the public and the collection of confidential health information. Personal health information about an individual includes identifying information about the individual that is not necessarily personal health information, but it is contained in a record that contains personal information about an individual such as the client's chart, medical history and any medical information. PHIPA act came into force on November 1, 2004. The Act has two parts: The Personal Health Information Protection Act (PHIPA) and The Quality-of-Care Information Protection Act.

Ontario's Personal Health Information Protection Act, 2004(PHIPA) sets out legal obligations for health information custodians, including dentists, to ensure that the privacy of their patients' personal health information is protected. A dentist is responsible for ensuring that all staff and other agents acting on their behalf are aware of requirements for maintaining confidentiality with respect to a patient's personal health information. Specifically, a dentist is responsible for ensuring that they only collect, use and disclose personal health information with the consent of the patient or as permitted or required by PHIPA.

A dentist is also responsible under PHIPA to take steps that are reasonable in the circumstances to ensure that records of personal health information in their custody or control are retained, transferred and disposed of in a secure manner. In particular, health information custodians must ensure that records of personal health information in their custody or control are protected against theft, loss and unauthorized use or disclosure, and to ensure that the records containing the information are protected against unauthorized copying, modification or disposal. Compliance with PHIPA

Ontario dentists must adhere to several aspects of PHIPA. The Ministry of Health and Long-

Term Care issued a checklist to assist health care providers in meeting the legislation's initial requirements, which can be found as part of the RCDSO's guide to compliance with PHIPA.

Important facts about PHIPA
- The act provides individuals with a right of access to personal health information about themselves, subject to limited and specific exceptions set out in the Act.
- As per the act the confidentiality of the information and the privacy of individuals must be protected while facilitating the effective provision of health care.
- It establishes rules for the collection, use and disclosure of personal health information about individuals.
- The act provides independent review and resolution of complaints with respect to personal health information.

PIPEDA - Personal Information Protection and Electronic Documents Act
PIPEDA defines personal information as "information about an identifiable individual" that includes any factual or subjective information, recorded or not, in any form. The Act, based on ten privacy principles developed by the Canadian Standards Association, is overseen by the Privacy Commissioner of Canada and the Federal Court. PIPEDA and PHIA are both pieces of legislation that establish rules to govern the collection, use and disclosure of personal information. PIPEDA – the Personal Information and Electronic Documents Act – came into force in 2001 and is a federal government initiative. While PIPEDA focuses on the privacy of information, it does not comprehensively cover those actions that are associated with the provision of health care. A great deal of information is now communicated and transmitted electronically. PIPEDA is an act that protects personal information in the hands of private sector organizations and provides guidelines for the collection, use and disclosure of that information in the course of commercial activity.

Important facts about PIPEDA
Under PIPEDA, dental offices are required to "destroy, erase or render anonymous information that is no longer required for an identified purpose or for a legal requirement." PHIA adds the necessity of having a written retention & destruction schedule for personal health information.

Under PIPEDA:
Personal information must be collected with informed consent and for a reasonable purpose
Personal information must be used and disclosed for the limited purpose for which it was
Personal information must be collected accurately and for genuine purpose
Personal information must be accessible for inspection and correction purpose

Personal information must be stored securely.

Dental Records and Patients

Patients are entitled to copies of any or all of their dental records. If a patient and/or authorized representative requests a copy of the patient's complete file this information must be provided. In most cases, a parent can request and obtain copies of the dental records for children who are under the age of 16 years. While a patient may request copies of the dental records for a spouse or a child 16 and over, the dentist will require the consent of these individuals to release their records.

As per Royal College of Dental Surgeons of Ontario, the request for dental records does not have to originate from another dental office, and dentists can provide copies of dental records to their patients directly if requested. The requests made by patients and the release of dental records should be documented in the patients' records. The release and transfer of dental records should be accomplished within one to two weeks of receipt of the request. Whether this is possible may depend on the number and type of dental records requested and whether the services of an outside duplication facility (for dental radiographs and study models) are required.

Privacy Officer and Dental office administration

A Privacy Officer is a designate at your office who is responsible for ensuring that any inquiries, complaints and concerns are responded to in a prompt and appropriate manner Client charts and other patient personal information are considered part of the client's confidential record and must be handled and processed accordingly. It is the responsibility of the health care provider and Dental Office Administrator to protect the personal health information contained in the charts while treating clients and exercising sensitivity to privacy. Should a client have questions or concerns about the privacy of their information, they should be directed to the Privacy Officer. The Privacy Officer will be responsible for responding to client concerns in a timely manner and provide copies of the Privacy Code available upon request.

CHAPTER 28
DENTIST – PATIENT/CLIENT RELATIONSHIP

A positive and professional relationship between a patient and their dentist is critical to the success of diagnosis and treatment. Dentists have an obligation to develop, maintain and foster a successful relationship with their patient.

Continuous and Preventive dental care

Continuum of care includes referrals, recalls, and other follow-up on treatment initiated at your clinic. Many patients need specialty care such as oral surgery, molar root canals, periodontal surgery, orthodontics, and specialized paediatric dental procedures. If your clinic does not provide these services, this does not relieve you of the responsibility of helping patients obtain them. You may refer them to the other dentists/specialist dentistry practices for their treatments.

Preventive dental services include routine oral examinations, X-rays, cleanings, pits and fissure sealants, and fluoride treatments. Educational instruction such as proper brushing and flossing methods is also considered the best way to prevent tooth decay.

Using different software in electronic dental records maintenance systems, you can set up continuing care types that tell you how often patients should be seen for certain procedures, such as prophylaxis or preventive care, X-rays, restorations or scaling. When you schedule appointments for the procedures attached to those continuing care types, the software automatically adds those patients to the continuing care schedule.

Important points related to spectrum of dental Care for clients
- Try to provide the best variety of dental care at your dental practice.
- Patient needing any service/treatment not available at your place, provide suitable referral.
- For the service referral not available at your clinic, document that the referral was made; or, if the patient refuses the referral, document the refusal too.
- Keep records of consultations and reports from the professionals to whom you refer patients.
- For any dental service requiring any form of follow-up, keep records of how that follow-up was provided.

- If patients miss appointments and fail to complete an agreed-upon course of treatment, document all of your attempts to re-appoint the patient and complete the treatment as per the plan.
- For any biopsy or laboratory work performed in your clinic, keep records of where the specimen was sent, the report from the pathologist, and the notification of the patient of the results of the biopsy and any further treatment recommended.
- If a patient requires services outside your scope of care but cannot afford them, you may refer them to local/provincial health departments, dental schools, or other agencies where they can get appropriate and affordable treatments and also document your all efforts you made.

Patients' Rights and the Canadian Health Care System

The delivery of health care in Canada has always been a mixture of public and private providers. While 70% of the total cost of health care is covered by public insurance, there has always been a strong role played by private out-of-pocket and employer-based insurance for services not covered publicly, such as dentistry and nonsurgical vision care (Sanmartin et al., 2014).

Dental services provided by dentists in their offices are not included in the public funding envelope; however, some dental services provided in hospitals are covered under insurance. It is important to note that public dental services represent a very small proportion of the overall dental services in Canada.

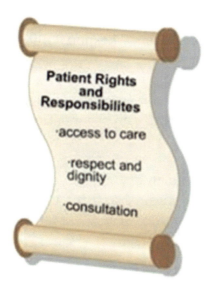

PATIENTS' BILL OF RIGHTS

When discussing patients' rights in the context of the Canadian health care system, it is important to distinguish between "collective" rights and "individual" rights and entitlements.

• Collective rights- are broad principles relating to the general societal obligation to make reasonable access to health care available for the entire population. What is reasonable in terms of the number and range of provided services depends on political, social and economic factors.

• Individual rights and entitlements-are what individuals are entitled to and can expect at various stages of the health care system when they interact with health care providers and institutions. These rights include rights to information, privacy, confidentiality, and consent to treatment.

The rights and responsibilities of patients are often combined into one document. A "Patient's Bill of Rights and Responsibilities" should be made available to patients in the form of posters conspicuously displayed in the clinic or as pamphlets or flyers.

Patients' Rights
- Access to care
- Respect and dignity
- Privacy and confidentiality
- Personal safety
- Staff identification by name and title
- Communication
- Consent
- Consultation
- Refusal of treatment
- Continuity of care
- Clinic rules and regulations Patients' Responsibilities
- Provision of accurate information
- Compliance with instructions
- Observance of hospital rules and regulations
- Respect and consideration of staff and other patients

CANADA HEALTH ACT

From the federal perspective, the primary objective of Canadian health care policy – to protect, promote and restore the physical and mental well-being of residents of Canada and to facilitate reasonable access to health services without financial or other barriers – is outlined in the Canada Health Act.

The fundamental collective principles underlying the Canadian health care system are set out in the five program criteria found in the Act as follows:

• **public administration-** ensures that the health care insurance plan of each province is administered and operated on a non-profit basis by a public authority that is responsible to the provincial government.

- **Comprehensiveness-** means that each provincial health insurance plan must cover all "insured health services," provided by hospitals, medical practitioners, or dentists or similar or additional services rendered by other health care practitioners where permitted.
- **Universality-** each provincial health insurance plan must cover all persons resident in a province.
- **Portability-** means that residents moving to another province must continue to be covered for insured services by the home province during a minimum waiting period
- **Accessibility-** means that insured health services should be provided on uniform terms and conditions and on a basis that does not impede or preclude reasonable access to those services.

Follow-up instructions for patients

A dental follow up is a crucial way to continue to build trust and loyalty from a patient. Studies show that patients recall less than one-half of verbal instructions after 24 hours. Unclear instructions after treatment and post-operative complications are two common sources of patient confusion and dissatisfaction. Some patients experience post-operative anxiety and may lead to unnecessary follow-up visits. Some patients fail to follow post-operative instructions or to report significant post-operative symptoms, consequently creating problems that could easily have been prevented.

Tips on Developing Follow-Up Instructions

- It is good to figure out the best way to follow up with your patient. It's good to follow up when they don't have another appointment.
- Instructions must be written in easy-to-understand, non-technical terms, preferably in the patient's own language.
- Instructions should begin with an explanation of the procedure and should describe what the patient needs to do and what to avoid.
- Instructions should include the normal responses to the treatment such as mild swelling, pain or jaw muscle soreness the first post operative night.
- Instructions should include a list of unpleasant outcomes such as fever or prolonged bleeding that should warrant immediate notification of the clinic.
- Clear and brief patient education sheets can help you to avoid post-operative problems to the patients and contribute to informed consent.
- You should provide the patient a telephone number for contact after hours.
- You can send out a generic and impersonal letter, email or message asking your patients to call your office.
- You may also follow up with your patient by calling him/her and have a personal conversation with them about the appointment they need.

DENTISTRY AS A BUSINESS

Since in the modern era, dental offices have become larger and more complex, there is increased competition in the marketplace. Clients of dental services are more aware of the health and esthetic benefits that can be achieved through dental services, and they have higher expectations in service excellence. There is a mutual relationship between the health care provider and the dental clients, who are informed consumers and active participants in their own wellness.

Customer care in Dentistry and the Business of Relationships

Dentistry is a relationship business. Customer service is critical in dentistry. Clients arrive at your office as informed consumers who have high expectations and little tolerance for delay. As a Dental Office Administrator how you communicate with your clients and each other is what creates the atmosphere for the office and sets the stage for your practice success. If your client/patient service skills are slow or sloppy, clients can take their business elsewhere. Without dental clients, you do not have a business. As a Dental Office Administrator, your communications should reflect your mutual commitment to wellness and client comfort by always presenting a positive and professional image of you and your dental practice.

The Role of The Office Administrator

The Dental Office Administrator (DOA) is the link between the clinical expertise of the dental providers to the dental consumer (the client). As a dental office administrator, you are the first point of contact with your clients. Your first impression is very important while dealing with the clients for the success of your dental practice. Customer service in dentistry is critical because it secures your future in business. Gaining clients and keeping them are your only source of revenue generating activities, everything else generates expense. It is the role of the dental office administrator to ensure that breakdowns do not occur. The Dental Office Administrator (DOA) must make it sure that a client should never leave your office unhappy or dissatisfied with the service he/she received.

Dental Office Administrators face many of the complex issues such as the changes in privacy laws, insurance adjudication, personnel performance issues, client relations, marketing and advertising and many other. As a Dental Office Administrator, you are the most watched person in the group and your behavior influences everyone else. You are required to lead by example and establish leadership influence by always displaying a mature attitude and treating people fairly. Your personal influence as a team leader grows when you behave the way that you expect team members to behave. When everyone feels involved in the success of the practice, you have formed a group of people who want to be part of the team and have you leading as a dental office administrator.

Some of the duties of the Dental Office Administrator:

- patient and staff communications
- patients scheduling
- staff scheduling
- coordinate regular meetings
- preparing and maintaining personnel records
- make effective financial arrangements with clients
- hiring and termination of staff
- prepare and conduct performance reviews
- continuing care systems
- handling and controlling the office budget
- responsible for accuracy of financial transactions related to Accounts Receivable and Accounts Payable
- report to the doctor(s) on regular basis.
- In brief, a Dental Office Administrator is responsible for coordinating the daily activities of the dental team to ensure that the office runs efficiently and effectively.

Required skills of a Dental Office Administrator:
- to work independently and efficiently
- to effectively use communication skills for clients and staff
- to use interpersonal skills effectively to build and maintain working relationships
- to drive your dental team to perform efficiently
- to work under pressure
- to delegate duties to others
- to keep the team focused and on track
- to problem solve
- to effectively manage stress
- to motivate staff
- to handle matters and think critically
- to be available where needed
- to be a positive role model to staff
- to give and take feedback in a positive manner and direction
- to hire and orient new staff
- to perform staff performance reviews
- to design and implement new marketing ideas
- to monitor case presentations and promote case acceptance
- Meet regularly to pull the team together to set plans
- to monitor and critically analyze patient feedback
- to follow-up with referrals

Important points for managing client complaints:

- Be professional, be understanding and be patient
- Don't make it a prestige issue
- Ask the client/patient how the situation developed
- Listen carefully to what the client/patient is saying
- Be tactful and avoid embarrassing the client/patient.
- Give the client/patient the benefit of the doubt
- Let the client/patient vent before attempting to deal with the problem
- Acknowledge their feelings and apologise for the inconvenience
- Show the client/patient that you care about, how they feel, and you are doing your best to help them
- Solve the problem, or find someone who can help in the matter amiably

Challenges in the patient-dentist relationship

From time to time, challenges may arise in the patient-dentist relationship. Dentists are expected to make a concerted effort to solve problems and rebuild relationships. If those efforts fail, a formal and respectful process must be followed to end the relationship must be followed. If the dentist-patient relationship is no longer co-operative and trusting, or if it becomes antagonistic, it may be best for the parties to go their separate ways. If a dentist feels that dismissal is the best option, the patient should be notified formally, preferably in writing. Letters should be sent by the dentist or in the dentist's name.

If the patient ends the relationship for any reason, you should:
- Document the patient's decision in your record
- Advise the patient in writing of incomplete treatment plans
- Recommend continuation of unfinished treatment
- Offer to forward records to the patient's next dentist
- Document these steps in the patient's record.

A certified letter is not necessary if the clinic closes. However, you should still provide the patient reasonable advance written notice, at least 30 days, that the relationship will be ending. You should also inform the patient how to seek the care of another dentist in the area, provide information regarding emergency care, and include advice for future treatment, if necessary.

CHAPTER 29
DENTAL OFFICE
PATIENT APPOINTMENT SYSTEM

I t is very vital to have a good appointment system in place for a successful and efficient dental practice. The appointment system for a dental practice contains lists of all the scheduled patients and events for the dentist and the staff. The appointment system is the control centre of the dental office and an important factor in the success or failure of a dental practice. The practice should be controlled through the appointment system but not by it. A dentist needs to decide if patients are going to be seen at the clinic by appointment, on a walk-in basis, or both. Part of the decision is based on the mission of the dental office. For example, if the mission is to alleviate pain and suffering, then a walk-in system may serve your needs. If, however, one wants to provide more comprehensive levels of care, then an appointment system will be necessary.

Performance of most dental procedures requires predictable amounts of time. Since specific instruments and materials are required for different procedures, appointment planning helps clinic staff plan operatory set up and sterilization procedures in an efficient and timely manner. All dentists are different, but most regular check-ups should be uneventful, and therefore pretty short.

According to a survey conducted by the American Dental Association, the average length of an appointment with a general practitioner is 52.1 minutes. However, with a specialist (such as an orthodontist), that number may drop a bit to about 30-40 minutes per appointment. Overall, it believed that any dental-related appointment should last an average of 50.7 minutes. Hence, it is advisable to ask the patient/client to budget about an hour or so for the treatment.

A comprehensive dental exam is the first appointment that most patients will receive. Future appointments can then be scheduled for discrete amounts of time based on the treatment plan. Multiple procedures or "quadrant" dentistry can be planned with each patient's care delivered in the fewest possible number of appointments. Quadrant dentistry means that all the dental treatment required in a quadrant is carried out in a single appointment. This is perceived as convenient for some dentists and some patients, as fewer appointments are required overall.

Dental practice management

An efficient arrangement for any dental office staff would be to have one person designated as the dental scheduling administrator/ coordinator. Another dental office administrator can possibly be assigned as the financial coordinator for an efficient management system in the office. With this arrangement, each staff person can be held accountable for specific assignments, such as scheduling and business collections. Job performance, whether good or bad, can then be measured by the amount of downtime (5% or less) and the percentage of collection (a goal of 96% or more).

It is important to know that poor management of the appointment system can result in great pressure, increasing stress and tension among staff members, and it can turn the reception room into a waiting room of discontented patients. This may lead to reduced productivity and increased chances of financial loss and harmony at workplace. Hence, everyone in the staff of a dental office should analyze the practice on the regular basis and determine an organized system of appointment control that maximizes productivity, reduces staff tension, and maintains concern for patients' needs.

APPOINTMENT-MANAGEMENT

Important points for Efficient Appointment Management

1. Put one person in charge of the appointment system.
2. In a traditional appointment book, make accurate and neat entries.
3. Accommodate the patient as much as possible but maintain control of the appointment schedule.
4. Always have a patient being treated in each dental chair.
5. Avoid scheduling repetitive procedures over long periods.
6. Be aware of production goal criteria.
7. Schedule the workload according to the staff members' body clocks.
8. Assign clinical tasks only to legally qualified personnel.
9. Avoid leaving large blocks of time between appointments.
10. Establish guidelines for problem situations.
11. Make sure that the practice is controlled through the appointment system rather than by it.

Appointment Time Schedule and important points to consider while Scheduling

• The dental office administrators must deal with a variety of situations when scheduling dental appointments.

• Time allocation for each type of treatment should be determined by the staff and a template provided so that all those responsible for appointment management understand the number of units that need to be scheduled for each type of treatment.

• Remember not all patients are same. Hence, time duration may need to modify depending upon the individual requirement and situation. An average amount of time for each type of procedure should be determined, though. In case of a complex procedure, the dentist needs to identify this with the office administrator so that a time adjustment in appointment can be made.

• The management of the dental appointment book requires a well-defined treatment plan, an established appointment sequence, and an ability to maintain strict control over the appointment book while still meeting the needs of patients.

• Generally, the same type of treatment should take the same amount of time (e.g., a full gold crown preparation on a molar may take a dentist two or three units, 30 to 45 minutes, depending on the type of unit). However, some modification in the plan may be anticipated in certain situations.

• After the average time is determined for a variety of services provided, then a schedule can be designed and provided to the entire staff so that everyone is familiar with time allocations.

• Consideration should be given to the time needed to clean and prepare a treatment room when making patient schedule and chair availability.

• Computer software must be updated and so are the regular patients details in the software.

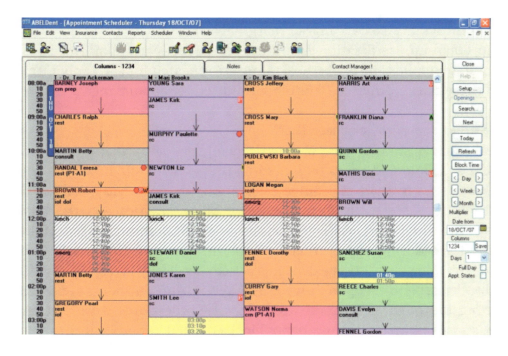

Walk-in patients in Dentistry

A walk-in dental clinic is the one where the dental services are available day and night to help patients with their dental issues. If anyone has chipped a tooth during a physical activity or damaged portions of their teeth after an accident, they can rely on a walk-in dental clinic to offer quality and professional dental services. These services also include emergency dental services. Care for walk-in patients is targeted to their chief complaint, so is usually unpredictable and frequently more time-consuming. Walk-in dental services, however, depends on the dentist. While some providers do accept walk-ins, a lot of well-established dentists prefer to work by appointment only.

The dental administrator should be able to establish the nature of the complaint, obtain appropriate radiographs and other studies (e.g., blood pressure, blood glucose level, diabetes, or other disease condition, if any) before determining what services are needed for that visit. Following this, the operatory be set up for the needed procedure. However, the provision of multiple procedures or quadrant dentistry at each visit is generally unfeasible with a walk-in system.

In establishing an appointment system, clinic administrators will need to decide on the style of practice that they wish to promote. Longer appointments with multiple procedures per visit promote comprehensive care and the completion of treatment plans as quickly as possible. Shorter appointments with few procedures per visit focus on seeing the greatest number of people possible. In making this decision, the following points should be considered:

• Short appointments usually mean that only one (or 2 at the most) procedures are completed at each visit.
• Short appointments also have higher marginal costs.
  o Set-up, Clean-up, Sterilization time are repeated for each appointment.
  o Disposable supplies and anaesthesia time are repeated for each appointment.
  o All of these can account for 10 or more minutes per appointment.

How should appointments be scheduled?

Each dental practice should have a dental scheduling administrator/coordinator who maintains the schedule and keeps patients in a proper schedule flow. In a dental practice in which there is more than one office assistant with no exactly defined duties, these administrators are likely to perform the same basic functions in the business office, such as answering the phone, collecting money, patient communication, filing, verifying insurance, and scheduling appointments. Appointment scheduling will depend on the number of chairs and providers the dental practice has. A day is usually divided into 10 or 15-minute blocks, depending upon the type of practice. Appointments are scheduled for the appropriate number of these blocks to accommodate procedures. Administrators with the help of dentists can estimate the number of blocks needed per procedure or visit, including the time needed to set up, clean and disinfect the dental operatory.

As the number of chairs and providers increases, the complexity of scheduling also increases. An efficient appointment system should keep all the dental operatories occupied during the day, without making patients wait or staff rush. This balance may not be easy to achieve, though. There is no single best answer for how to schedule appointments, per se. It is advisable to consult with a practice management specialist or use the expertise of experienced staff to set up the system. In the present times, different types of Dental Practice Management Software Packages are very helpful in managing the appointment system in most of the dental practices at provincial and national levels.

Important points related to Scheduling appointments

- Most practice management specialists recommend that for the better practice management, appointments should be scheduled no more than 2 and one-half to 3 weeks in advance.
- Special considerations must be made for multi-appointment procedures such as root canals, surgeries or crown and bridge to be completed properly with due care.
- Incidence of broken appointments can increase when appointments are scheduled more than three weeks in advance.
- If appointments need to be scheduled more than three weeks out, then carry out either a mailed or phone-based reminder system.
- Managing the appointment book in proper manner requires that the clinic regularly define, and track completed treatment plans.
- You should avoid the appointments to be scheduled more than two months in advance.
- Rescheduling patients beyond time frame is inappropriate and is inconsistent with quality clinical care. Hence, many clinics keep few times in a week per month or certain times each day unscheduled or lightly scheduled to use for rescheduling patients or to handle emergencies.

A broken or missed appointments

A broken appointment is when you cancel or reschedule an appointment with less than 48-hour notice or do not show up for the scheduled appointment. Most dental practices get affected adversely by broken or missed appointments. Down time negatively impacts productivity in the practice but can be minimized by maintaining a list of patients who have indicated they are available on short notice for appointments.

Many dental clinics choose to not have a broken appointment policy because of the barriers faced by some of their patients such as unforeseen circumstances, not having transportation, inclement weather, erratic traffic conditions or unpredictable or inflexible work schedules.

Prevention of missed/broken Appointments

The Dental Office Administrator (DOA) can select or develop their own methods to deal with missed/broken appointments in dental practice. They can select the combination of methods that works best for their particular circumstances.

- The practice/DOA can develop a customised policy for missed/broken Appointments and universally enforce it.

- They can make a signed contract with all clients about their rights and responsibilities and implement the contract.
- Confirm all appointments, including recall and hygiene appointments, the day before the appointment
- It should be enforced that all patients come in and complete all registration paperwork before they are given their first appointment to prevent missing their exam appointment.
- The policy may emphasise that patients must call in and confirm their own appointments the day before their visit or may lose the appointment.
- Decrease the amount of time that the clinic is fully scheduled in advance.
- emergency patients after the completion of their emergency visit can be asked to call back in a day or two to schedule an exam appointment.
- Some clinics become successful in reducing missed/broken appointments by requiring patients with missed appointments to write a letter to the clinic manager/DOA detailing the reason for the missed the appointment and why they should be given the next appointment.

Dental Appointment Agreement

It is important for patients to keep their dental appointments, because missed/broken appointments result in lost time and revenue for the dental practice where time is money.

Rescheduling Appointments

As a DOA you know that sometimes situations need rescheduling of clients' appointments and you may explain the details to the client as mentioned below.

<u>**Sample of Dental Appointment Agreement**</u>

If you need to reschedule, please call our clinic as soon as you know that you will not be able to keep the appointment, preferably at least 24 hours before the appointment time.

If you miss a scheduled appointment or cancel it at the last minute, a broken appointment will be recorded in your dental chart.

If you are more than 10 minutes late for an appointment, a missed appointment will also be recorded, and you may have to be rescheduled if there is not enough time to complete your procedure.

If you have 2 missed appointments during the past 6 months, you will not be able to make a regular appointment for a period of 6 months from the date of the second missed appointment. You are still eligible for emergency dental care during that time.

I understand the Dental Appointment Agreement and agree to follow the terms of the missed/ broken appointment policy.

_____

Patient Name (please print)   *Date*

_____

Patient or Guardian Signature

Handling dental emergencies

Dental emergencies such as toothaches, abscess, excruciating pain or broken fillings are common in dental offices. Preventing dental injuries is as important to good oral health as regular visits to the dentist and personal dental care such as brushing and flossing. Many dental practices make time available for emergencies by keeping one or more appointment slots open each day until 24 hours in advance of the appointment time. If no one calls for an emergency visit, then the appointment can be scheduled for a regular patient. Failure to accommodate patients of record with urgent needs, especially if those needs are post-operative problems from services that your clinic provided, can lead to charges of patient abandonment.

Toothache or tooth pain is caused when the nerve root of a tooth is irritated. Tooth infection, decay, injury or loss of a tooth are the most common causes of dental pain. Patients must be explained the following simple tips in case of emergency situations:

- Explain your symptoms to DOA and ask to be seen as soon as possible.
- There is no one-size-fits all approach to oral health treatment and pain management.
- Over-the-counter medicines, like ibuprofen and acetaminophen can be effective for temporary pain relief. Ease the pain with an over-the-counter pain medicine that works for you. Please check you don't have any allergic reaction with any OTC or other medications. You must inform your DOA and dentist earliest possible.
- However, never put medication directly against the gums near an aching tooth as it may burn gum tissue.
- You may hold an ice pack against your face at the spot of the sore tooth if it relieves the pain.
- Never use a heating pad, hot water bottle or any other source of heat on your jaw. Heat will make things worse instead of better.

How to handle dental emergency patients:

- Ask emergency patients to call back for their follow-up exam and treatment, rather than providing an appointment at the conclusion of the emergency visit.
- After emergency patients call back for a follow-up appointment, an exam and basic preventive and restorative treatment should be provided prior to more complex treatment such as root canal treatment (RCT), crowns, bridges, and removable prosthetics.

- In general, perform the essential emergency treatment at the time of emergency visit whenever possible, rather than providing only pain medication and/or antibiotics asking the patient to return on another day.

CHAPTER 30
DENTAL BILLING & INSURANCE

Billing of the patient services is one of the important tasks of Dental Administrative office. Dental office and the administrators should be clear, open and upfront about the actual costs that are involved with any treatment plan. Dentists have a legal and ethical obligation to obtain their patients' informed consent prior to the start of treatment. This means discussing the proposed treatment and sharing risks and other information before the patient agrees to proceed, including treatment costs.

Dental care coverage by province
Depending on patient/client eligibility, each province has their own government dental programs.

- **Alberta** offers multiple programs for low-income residents ranging from children to adults. Alberta dentists provide dental services at reduced fees for Albertans through various social programs offered by the Government of Alberta.
- **British Columbia** offers basic dental coverage for adults on income or disability assistance and for youth under 19 years old in families on assistance. Under dental coverage, basic dental costs are covered. Everyone who receives assistance can access emergency dental services to relieve pain.
- **Manitoba** has a provincial health plan called Manitoba Health, Seniors and Active Living. Under the health plan, some dental procedures are covered when performed in a hospital.
- **New Brunswick** offers a dental program to those who are over 19 years old who have special needs and qualify for assisted health care. Exams, x-rays, dentures and fillings are covered. This Health Services Dental Program assists clients of this department who are over the age of 19 with coverage for specific dental benefits that are not covered by other agencies or private health insurance plans.
- **Newfoundland and Labrador** has multiple dental health plans for kids, young adults and adults. Each program offers different services and eligibility varies. The Children's Dental Health Program provides universal access to eligible dental services for children aged 12 years and under. The Income Support Program provides 'Basic Services' only, as listed in the Dental Health Plan Payment Schedule.
- **Northwest Territories** offers a school-based Oral Health Program to children attending

school to teach about oral health education and provide oral examinations. The Extended Health Benefits for Seniors Program provides those 60 years of age and over, who are non-Aboriginal and Métis, residents access to a range of dental benefits not covered by insurance. These visiting clinics are available to all NWT residents, and offer a wide variety of dental and hygienist services.

• **Nova Scotia** Children's Oral Health Program is for all children 14 years of age and under with a valid health card number. Once a year, children are able to have services such as one routine dental exam, one fluoride application and two x-rays.

• **Nunavut** offers an Oral Health Program to children in grade 7 and under. Children enrolled in the program are eligible for free dental screenings. Program services are provided by Dentists, Dental Therapists, Dental Hygienists, Territorial Community Oral Health Coordinators and Community Oral Health Coordinators.

• In **Ontario**, Healthy Smiles Ontario is a free dental program that includes regular check-ups, preventive care, and treatment for children and youth 17 and under. Ontario offers a few different programs for low income and/or disabled youths and seniors on income assistance or disability assistance. Children and youth currently receiving care from the programs listed above were automatically transitioned into the new Healthy Smiles Ontario program. Ontarians who qualify can access a variety of health care services in their community. There is also Cleft Lip and Palate/Craniofacial Dental Program for those who are eligible.

• **Prince Edward Island** -Dental Public Health provides preventative and treatment services to children 3-17 years of age. Dental treatment services are limited to children who are not covered by private dental insurance. Some dental care is also offered to long-term care residents. To access any of the services, an active PEI Health Card is required. Adults in long-term care facilities are provided with long-term care dental treatment, such as annual screenings for oral disease, cleaning and scaling.

• **Quebec** health insurance covers certain oral surgery. There are also services covered for children under age 10, including x-rays, fillings and tooth extractions. Dentists and denturists participating in the public plan render certain covered services. Children under age 10 and recipients of last-resort financial assistance may receive several services at no cost.

• **Saskatchewan** health coverage doesn't cover routine dental services. However, it does cover surgery related to accidents and/or infection, extracting teeth and dental implants. Qualified individuals are eligible for a number of health services and products in addition to the universal health benefits.

• **Yukon** has Children's Dental Program, which provides services to newborns to grade 8 or grade 12, depending on place of residence. Services include diagnosis, preventative and restorative services.

Dental treatment in Ontario

Fees & Charges Regulatory body

Royal College of Dental Surgeons of Ontario (RCDSO) is the regulatory body for dentists in Ontario. It sets and enforce standards and provide leadership and education to the dental profession. According to RCDSO, Dentists have a legal and ethical obligation to obtain their patients' informed consent prior to the start of treatment. This means discussing the proposed treatment and sharing risks and other information before the patient agrees to proceed, including treatment costs. The Ontario Dental Association publishes a suggested fee guide for Ontario dentists. Dentists must tell patients if they intend to charge fees that are above the fees listed in the guide.

RCDSO Standards and recommendations to dentists

•   Estimates should include the cost of additional expense of materials (at cost) and laboratory fees (at cost), when applicable, and any additional treatment.

•   Dentists may provide estimates that include a range of low and high costs. In complex cases, they may discuss the costs of subsequent treatment.

•   Patients can and should ask questions to fully understand the proposed treatment and its associated costs. You may need to book a separate appointment to discuss the fees associated with a complex treatment plan.

•   A dentist should only proceed with treatment once informed consent is obtained. If a dentist determines that an alteration to the treatment plan is necessary during treatment, while the patient is in the chair, the dentist should explain the additional costs and confirm that the patient, parent or substitute decision maker agrees before proceeding.

•   Dentists should be clear, open and upfront about the actual costs that are involved with any treatment plan. If you have dental coverage and want predetermination of coverage, the dental office may prepare it for you. The office may discuss payment of costs or services not covered by insurance plans.

ODA Suggested Fee Guide

The Ontario Dental Association publishes The ODA Suggested Fee Guide for dentists which is based upon the provision of dental services which are performed under normal conditions. It is intended to serve only as a reference for the general practitioner to enable development of a structure of fees which is fair and reasonable to the patient and to the practitioner. The Guide is not mandatory, and each practitioner is expected to determine independently the fees which will be charged for the services performed. That means the fees may vary both above and below the Guide.

The Guide is not available on the ODA website. However, copies have been placed in the reference section of many public libraries so that members of the public can access this document. The Guide contains roughly 1,300 dental services and it is written using correct dental terminology.

Each dental service is identified by a five-digit number called a procedure code. The descriptions attached to the procedure code describe the dental service but not the reason the service was performed. For example, the Guide contains several procedure codes that describe veneers -- however, none of the descriptions identify the reason the veneer is being placed (i.e., for cosmetic reasons or to restore a tooth that is missing or has lost tooth structure). The Guide is a listing of dental services that general practitioners may perform. If the client has the procedure code for the treatment that was prescribed or performed by their dentist, they may contact the ODA's Practice Advisory Services staff who can provide with information about the suggested fees.

How Much Do Common Dental Procedures Cost?

There are so many different types of dental procedures available, and the cost associated with each varies quite a bit. Further, the same procedure may also vary based on location and dentist. That said, the following is a list of some of the more common dental procedures and the average cost for each:

Here are some average costs, in Canadian dollars, for common dental procedures:
- Large Tooth Filling: $325
- Small Tooth Filling: $80 (Silver Filling), or $200 (White Filling)
- Root Canal: $800 However, in general it may vary from $300 – $2,000 per tooth, depending on the exact type of tooth
- Dental Crown: $1425 (Gold), or $1625 (Porcelain)
- Dental Bonding: $450
- Invisalign Braces: $7,249
- Veneer: $1,750
- Adult Dental Exam: $133
- Child Dental Exam: $67
- Tooth Extraction: $136 (starting at)
- Dentures – $1,000 – $8,000
- Dental implants – $1,000 – $3,000 per tooth.
- Full-mouth implants – $24,000 – $100,000

In Canada, a single dental implant may cost between $900 to $3000. A full mouth reconstructive dental implant may cost up to $96,000.

OHIP and dental costs

Ontario Health Insurance Plan (OHIP) covers all Ontario residents, but only certain dental situations are fully covered. This could include oral surgery provided in a hospital and only in extreme situations, such as:
- Correcting birth defects
- Diseases of the jaw (tumors)
- Correcting jaw and face damage due to an accident

Above services are OHIP dental coverage, meaning dentists provide the service and bill

OHIP. However, OHIP dental coverage does not cover regular dental services, such as check-ups, scalings, x-rays and root canals/extractions.

Dental Fees vs Dental Plans

As explained by ODA (Ontario dental Association), there may be a difference between dentist's fees and the amount covered by a dental plan because for the following reasons:

I. The Factors Considered When Calculating the Cost

The amount a dentist may charge, and the amount client's dental plan may reimburse them for might be different because these two prices are not derived in the same way. When an employer and insurance carrier determine the amount of money a dental plan will pay for services covered under the plan, they take into account the specific circumstances of a company and its employees. The factors include company funds available for employee benefits, the nature and extent of use of the dental plan by the employees, and which version of the ODA Suggested Fee Guide for General Practitioners is used by the insurance carrier.

The ODA fee guide is a reference of suggested fees for dental services that is updated annually by the Ontario Dental Association. Some employers may use a current issue of the guide, while others may use past issues of the guide. Most dentists set their own fees structure, considering the factors affecting both the practice and the patients served. The ODA Suggested Fee Guide helps dentists derive fees, but this is only a guide, and the fees are only "suggested."

A dentist may use ODA Fee guide to formulate a fee for their dental services. Once a dentist has established a fee for a certain service, with special exceptions, he/she will charge that fee to all patients, regardless of whether or not the patient has a dental plan.

II. The Plan Design

For some dental services, payment may be based on a cost-sharing arrangement between the employer and employee. In these cases, the patient pays for a portion of the cost, while the plan pays for the remainder. As identified on the claim form when a client sign after receiving a service, they are responsible for the bill. This means he/she is also responsible to pay for the portion of the bill not covered by their plan - the portion known as the co-payment. It is illegal for the dentist to waive or ignore the co-payment and a dentist who does this could lose his or her licence.

III. The Individual Circumstances of the Patient

In case of any complex dental procedure/dental problem requiring lengthy or expensive dental services, the fee may be higher than the dentist's usual fee. Similarly, if the problem is less complex and requires less time or work to resolve, the fee may be lower than normal charges.

Sometimes due to unaffordability of costly treatment, a patient or group of patients refrain from obtaining even most required dental care. This can pose a great risk to patients who are in poor overall health, particularly those suffering from heart disease. For example, a toothache can result in oral infection and may be a higher health risk if not treated on time. In such situations, it is better to discuss the situation, including the fee and a better solution can be found rather than having the patient forgo the necessary care. This should involve working out financial terms with the dentist and discussing all possible options.

Dental Plans

Many Canadians may have a dental plan through their employer, union or provincial government. As a full partner in their own oral health care, every client has a right and responsibility to know how their dental plan works. Details of the plan and information can also be obtained from the service provider. It is also important to understand dental plan, especially someone is paying for dental care on their own.

Following are the key points related to dental plans:
- A dental plan and a treatment plan are two different things
- A dental plan is a means to help a client to pay for their dental treatment.
- Employers provide health and dental benefits for a variety of reasons, including the promotion of good health.
- A treatment plan is the personal plan a client and their dentist develop together to meet the client's oral health needs.
- Dental plan serves as a road map to good oral health and needed treatment should not be limited by what a dental plan will cover.

Types of dental insurance coverage

Each dental insurance plan will be different in what services are offered, but there are generally basic plans as mentioned below that insurance companies offer. These plans might vary slightly from insurer to insurer, so it's best to find out what exactly each plan covers.
- **Basic:** Most plans include basic services such as routine cleaning, exams and x-rays. The frequency that the insurer will pay for treatments varies for each plan. Some cover a routine exam every 6 months, while others every 9 or 12 months.
- **Comprehensive basic:** This plan covers the same as the basic plans, but also include periodontal treatment, root canals and denture cleaning and more.
- **Major:** These plans help cover extensive treatment that basic and comprehensive basic don't cover, such as crowns, bridges and more. Major plans may have waiting period, though. The services need a client to be a policyholder for at least a minimum number of months, even up to 3 years.
- **Orthodontic:** It usually covers braces or some other type of alignment to straighten teeth and jaws. Just like major plans, orthodontic plans can also have a waiting period of up to three years.

Individual vs group dental insurance

Health insurance provided to employees by an employer or by an association to its members is called group coverage. Health insurance an individual buy on their own—not through an employer or association—is called individual coverage. Depending on how many employees there are, benefits covered by group and individual plans may be different. Individual insurance is covered for single people, couples, or families, while group insurance is referring to employee benefits that are purchased by companies for their employees. There are also some services that are add-ons to extend an insurance policy for both individual and group.

Dental insurance is a straightforward product that is either called individual insurance or group insurance. Each insurance package varies in price and coverage of dental services offered. Group insurance covers all members of a specific group and their eligible dependants. It is often offered through an employee benefits package or through membership in a professional association. For example, Ontario Blue Cross provides dental insurance to their clients for common dental treatments and oral surgery that OHIP does not cover for them. They mention that their health insurance plans have no deductible, making their coverage suitable for self-employed individuals and others who do not have group insurance through their employer. For a big or small businesses, many companies such as *Cigna, Chambers plan and Lewer Canada* provide group dental plans where the employers can find the right group medical and dental insurance, life, accident, disability coverage and flexible health spending accounts for their business.

It is important to note that group insurance usually covers the same benefits regardless of the individual and typically cannot be personalized.

If your employer doesn't offer group insurance, you may be able to purchase it through a professional association or an alumni association.

If your employer offers supplementary health and/or dental insurance as part of a benefits package, they will sometimes pay the premiums. If you have group insurance through an association, you will have to pay premiums yourself.

FREE DENTAL SERVICES

Healthy Smiles Ontario is one government program that offers free dental services to children and youth 17 years old and younger who come from low-income households.

The program includes regular visits to a licensed dental provider and covers the costs of treatment including:

> *check-ups*
> *cleaning*
> *fillings (for a cavity)*
> *x-rays*
> *scaling*
> *tooth extraction*
> *urgent or emergency dental care (including treatment of a child's toothache or tooth pain)*

Cosmetic dentistry, including teeth whitening and braces, are not covered by the

program.

There is also free dental care for seniors 65 years of age and older from low income households called the Ontario Seniors Dental Care Program. The program provides free routine visits while covering costs for services such as check-ups, repairing broken teeth, x-rays, removing teeth, treating pain and gum conditions.

Dental care isn't included in the Canada Health Act, and most residents who aren't eligible for free dental care, or don't get benefits through their employer, end up paying for services through private insurance or out of their own pocket.

Dental plan administrators

A dentist may offer payment plans, but not all dentists do. A payment plan spreads out the cost of a dental procedure over time such as fillings, root canal, set of dentures, etc. Some dentists' plans may require weekly payments; others may have monthly payments. Dental plan contracts are lengthy, complex documents that define what services are covered and under what circumstances those services are eligible for reimbursement. The employer enters into a dental plan contract with a third party that act as the plan administrator. Employers sponsor dental plans for a variety of reasons, including the promotion of good health, keeping their work force healthy and fit, and attracting and retaining top-notch employees. Your employer should provide the details of the dental plan that are easy to understand. It gives a brief overview of the services that are covered, limitations and exclusions, and the fee guide used to calculate benefits.

Dental plan administrators are contractually required to reimburse clients based upon the terms of the dental plan contract. This means that in some instances, necessary treatment may not be covered. Moreover, certain limitations such as frequency limitations — for example, "This service is covered once every three years" — are easily understood, while others are more complex, such as, "This service is covered only when there is evidence of recurrent decay or fracture". Certain terms must be understood and explained in proper way.

LIMITATIONS OF DENTAL PLANS

- It may be possible that a dental plan for a patient may not cover his/her all treatments.
- Depending on how much coverage and the type of coverage the patient may have, their plan might not cover all necessary treatments.
- Also, if the patient has already maxed out the yearly amount, or their dental plan is limited to a certain number of treatments per annum, some of their treatments may not be covered under the plan and they may have to pay upfront for those treatments.
- Although the dental plans are designed to help patients pay for their dental treatments, there are usually some limitations. Idealistically, dental insurance plans

would cover 100% of the costs for all dental treatments. But in such a plan, the patient may have to pay quite a more premium for their insurance plan.

Patients'/Clients' perspectives & Dental plans:

Since the dental treatments can be moderately expensive to very expensive, it is wise for a patient/client to find out if their dental plan will cover a specific dental treatment. Moreover, in order to avoid disappointment and to budget accordingly, it is essential to go over their dental plan to see what their insurance covers and what it doesn't cover. Predeterminations will be especially helpful for a patient/client to figure out if they can afford an expensive procedure, or if they should find out an alternative payment method.

The patient can contact his/her dentist/dental office in this regard. The dental office administrator can submit a predetermination to the patient's insurance company. The insurer will then send the client or their dental office the amount the client's dental plan will cover for the treatment/procedure.

Ideal dental care is based on a solid relationship between the dentist and the patient, without third party interference. When the payment comes from the client/patient, there is a clear statement that the dental practice's first loyalty goes to the client, and not the insurance company, and also it should show the dental team that they value the service they are providing to their clients.

DENTAL BILLING - direct payment

The patients who have to pay for an entire dental bill up-front, they know how expensive dental treatments can get. Unfortunately, this fear of high cost for dental work generally scares off patients from getting the treatments they require. Many times, the patients put off treatments or avoid their dentist altogether. Because of this, with the passage of time, their oral health will deteriorate, ending up with the situations where they will require the treatments that are more expensive than before. Even if a patient has dental insurance, paying out-of-pocket upfront can be stressful. Hence, to prevent the scaring off patients, many dental clinics regularly offer direct billing.

WHAT IS DIRECT BILLING? how direct insurance billing works

Advantages:

a. Direct insurance billing relieves the stress of having to pay for an entire dental bill upfront.

b. And it helps patients get the treatments they need before their dental problems worsen.

c. It avoids the stress of not having adequate dental coverage.

d. As a result of direct billing, the patient will only have to pay for the remaining difference that insurance plan doesn't cover.

e. Direct billing is a quick, convenient way to pay for visits to dentist, helping save on time and upfront costs.

f.   With direct billing, one can avoid having to pay for the whole amount up front, submit a claim on own, and wait for claim to be processed and reimbursed.

Process:

Direct billing refers to an electronic transaction between a dental clinic and patient's insurance provider. During a visit to dentist, the dental office will submit a dental claim electronically to insurer with the total cost of the dental procedures completed that day. After the claim is submitted, insurer will respond with an invoice explaining how much insurance plan will cover for dental treatment(s). And the insurance company will pay dentist directly for a percentage of the total cost. As a result of direct billing, the patient will only have to pay for the remaining difference that insurance plan doesn't cover.

INSURANCE COMPANIES PAYMENT & DENTAL PLANS- DETAILS
Dental Plans and Dentists
The Dentist's and DOAs' Responsibilities

As a dental office administrator, you are a partner in your clients 'oral health. All treatment and care decisions should be made by you and your dentist based upon your clients' actual needs, aside from their dental plan coverage. It is interesting that the most successful dental entrepreneurs have learned to master both the patient and client relationship.

Following are the important points related to the Dentist's and DOAs' Responsibilities:

•   The dentist, in accordance with the Regulated Health Professions Act and applicable regulations should provide the information on available treatment options appropriate to address clients' dental care needs, regardless of the nature and extent of their dental plan coverage.

•   The dentist also helps clients by supplying information required to enable them to receive benefits they may be entitled under their dental plan.

•   When a client visits their dentist, it is dentist/DOA's duty to explain them about their dental condition and guide them for the required treatment alternatives that coincide with client's need and not with what is covered under client's benefit plan.

•   Client's individual needs may often be different from what their plan covers. Hence, your dental treatment planning and care decisions regarding the patients should be made based upon your clients' actual needs and health benefits, and not merely upon their dental plan coverage.

Dental Office Administrator and Dental Insurance

Dental Office Administrator (DOA) plays vital role in assisting the clients in understanding their insurance benefits without assuming the role of an insurance plan administrator. Insurance companies cannot diagnose a client's condition or prepare a treatment plan, only a dental professional can. DOA plays an important role here. DOA must understand the dental practice must be patient centered and not insurance driven, and a dental insurance program is a contract between the client's employer and the insurance carrier, not between the insurance carrier and the dentist. DOA can understand and effectively communicate with the insured clients about their dental insurance plan, their design and how they will work in the best interest of their clients. As a DOA you must help your patients to understand their dental plans benefit, however, it is important to remember that you do not become their plan administrator.

DOA Role in service explanation

DOA can competently explain the different types of Services available and provided to the clients.

Diagnostic—includes radiographs, diagnostic study models, panoramic x-rays, bitewings, periapicals, etc.

General—anesthetic, general and conscious sedation, laboratory services

Preventive—recall appointments, prophylaxis, pits and fissure sealants, etc.

Restorative—fillings, crowns, etc.

Endodontics—root canal therapy, pulp treatment and associated treatment

Oral Surgery—extractions, complicated and uncomplicated surgery

Orthodontics—orthodontic bands, braces, fixed and removable appliances

Periodontics—scaling, root planning, surgical procedures, etc.

Prosthodontics- Removable—full and partial dentures, relines, etc.

Prosthodontics- Fixed bridges etc.

Dental plans are designed to help patients pay for their dental treatment. However, not all dental treatments are eligible or fully reimbursable. If the client's dental treatment is only partially covered, he/she will have to share in the cost of their dental care.

The Patient's Responsibilities

As per ODA (Ontario Dental Association), there are more than 30,000 dental plan contracts in Ontario, and each can be little different from the other.

Following are the important points related to the clients'/patients' Responsibilities:

• As a client, one should understand the details of dental plan, and to supply your dental plan administrator with necessary information such as pre-treatment forms, claim forms or any supplementary information.

• Patients are also responsible for making arrangements for payment to your dentist for the dental care received.

• patient must understand that dental services may appear expensive in Ontario and one may be accustomed to not paying for general health care for physical health problems. However, its important to comprehend the fact that the cost of providing dental health services is extremely high in this day and age.

- If patient consents to any dental procedures, it is patient's responsibility to pay on the day of service. It is the responsibility of the dental insurance carrier (a third party) to directly reimburse patient for the portion of the procedure that is covered.
- The actual contract is between patient, as the employee (and the employer) and the insurance company.
- Many make the mistake of believing that the contract is between the dentist and the insurance company, and that may lead to many misunderstandings.
- Patients have a right to go ahead or not with any recommended treatment.
- Patient's dental office will usually be happy to contact patient's insurer and gain information regarding patient's dental plan, benefits and percentage coverage. They can even submit pre-determinations or estimates of required future treatment and get a response of insurance responsibility for reimbursement to the patient, prior to treatment.
- Keep in mind that this is usually subject to a yearly maximum benefit amount and the year does not always begin on January 1.
- Eventually, it is patient's responsibility to understand patient's dental plan, coverage and to pay for patient's dental work.
- There are also many dental credit companies in existence and patient's dentist can advise patient as to the one that best suits patient's situation.
- If a patient is not covered for all necessary treatments, and if cost is a major concern, patient may talk to patient's dentist and see if some other kind of payment arrangement can be negotiated before starting the treatment.

Generally, majority of dentists accept payment from insurance companies under normal conditions. However, there are certain situations when many of the dentists prefer not to accept payment from insurance companies.

Riskes of Direct Insurance Billing

There are several risks involved for dentists who offer direct insurance billing, so some dentist may prefer to avoid these risks altogether. These risks include:

a. Dentists may not receive payments from insurance companies if there is an issue with the claim. There may be liability if there are problems with the claim. And dental clinics often won't find out if a claim is denied until later on once the patient has left.

b. Extra time and money spent on administrative duties.

c. Stressful, time-consuming audits. Insurance companies may audit dental providers who submit insurance claims.

d. Lengthy waits for reimbursements. Insurance companies can take up to 30 days to pay dentists, which can be too long of a time and cause cash-flow/payroll problems for some dentists.

e. Dental officers are required to stay up to date with the ever-changing claim policies.

Commercial Lab Charges

There are many dental services that require additional "commercial laboratory procedures." Dental procedures that involve the services of a commercial laboratory may include:

- dentures
- veneers, crowns, bridges
- inlays or onlays — small and large restorations, respectively
- posts and cores for crown and bridge restorations
- implant procedures
- night guards, sports guards, sleep apnea appliances, orthodontic appliances
- repairs to any of the above restorations or appliances.

Laboratory Fees

Dentists arrange for a commercial laboratory to do the work to precise specifications meeting clients' treatment needs. In most cases, the laboratory services are performed by companies and not the dentist. While the patients have to pay for the lab fee, it is not the dentist's fee. The fees charged for laboratory services are in addition to the dentist's professional fee for the service or treatment provided.

When completing the claim form, the fee for the service performed by the dentist, such as a crown or bridge, will be listed as a professional fee. The laboratory charges reported on the form, using procedure code 99111, will be the fee charged by the commercial laboratory.

Lab Fees and Dental Plan Coverage

Laboratory charges must be completed in conjunction with other services. The amount payable by client's dental plan will be limited to the reimbursement percentage of the services that required the lab work. This percentage is determined by the employer or plan sponsor and there are a variety of ways in which reimbursement is handled by the plan administrator.

To find out the level of reimbursement that can be expected from the dental plan, a client can request to their dentist to prepare an estimate of the professional services and the estimated laboratory charges, which should then be submitted to their plan administrator. The predetermination of benefits a client can receive back from their plan administrator will explain how their benefits for these services are calculated so that the clients are aware of their dental costs before receiving the treatment.

DENTAL INSURANCE, PREMIUM & CLAIM

Dental insurance is a type of health insurance designed to pay a portion of the costs associated with dental care. Dental insurance programs are designed by insurance carriers or companies and offered to the employers at diverse costs for the premiums, or monthly fees which the employer pay for the benefit. They are usually part of group benefits packages for employees. The employer selects a plan that best suitable to their requirements, while keeping the cost of the plan affordable. They usually prefer to select a plan design that is the least expensive and most appropriate for the group.

There are several different types of individual, family, or group dental insurance plans grouped into 3 basic categories: Indemnity (or sometimes called: true dental insurance) which allows you to see any dentist you want who accepts insurance, Preferred Provide Network dental plans (PPO; briefly discussed below), and dental Health Managed Organizations (DHMO) in which you are assigned to an in-network dentist or in-network dental office and must stay within that network to receive your dental benefits.

Most dental offices have a fee schedule, or a list of prices for the dental services or procedures they offer. Dental insurance companies have similar fee schedules which is generally based on Usual and Customary dental services, an average of fees in your area. When a dentist signs a contract with a dental insurance company that provider agrees to match the insurance fee schedule and give their customers a reduced cost for services, this is considered an *In-Network Provider or Participating Provider network (PPO)*.

Some of the features of dental insurance plans:
- Some dental insurance plans may have waiting periods. This is a period before certain benefits will be covered.
- Some plans may have an annual maximum benefit limit. Thus, once the annual maximum benefit is exhausted and additional treatments may become the patient's responsibility. Each year that annual maximum is reissued. The reissued date may vary as a calendar year, company fiscal year, or date of enrollment based on specific plan.
- Plans for orthodontics usually has a separate limit.
- Some plans may have an annual deductible depending on type of treatment rendered. After the deductible is met, the remaining dental plan benefit is paid at its specified percentage or fee schedule.

Selection of the right dental insurance for an individual depends on what is best suited for their needs and budget. For those with teeth and oral health in good standing, a basic plan may be suitable over a more comprehensive plan. Some plans might also have dental add-ons that one can pay extra for as the budget and needs change.

A *premium for a dental insurance* is the amount of money an individual or business pays for their dental insurance policy. Along with the selected package, different factors also come into play while calculating the premium. These include individual's age, dental records, and illness history. Other factors also affect the premium such as the location of their residence and how many dependents are in the family.

There are also Group benefits, also known as *employee benefits*. They are the part of the compensation package for employees to help cover some or all medical and dental costs. Each group benefit package is different in what is covered. Some benefit packages cover up to a certain fixed amount, while others cover up to a certain percentage. For example, one employer might cover up to 80% of basic dental procedures, while another employer might reimburse up to $500 or $ 700 for any dental work. Sometimes, employers also opt for specific add-ons to the existing coverage or let the employee personalize their benefits. Also, there are some private insurances to help bridge the gap of the employee benefits.

Part-time or contract employees generally are not eligible for benefits, so they may need to get private insurance or pay for any work out of their own pocket. For self-employed individuals, before deciding on getting insurance or not, they can make sure to know what is covered because not every plan has what they need. Some plans also come with yearly spending limitations or limiting procedures, such as only covering certain emergencies.

To claim dental benefits, a claim form must be completed and submitted to the claim provider. While submitting a claim to dental insurance providers, a specific process set out by the dental insurance provider need be followed. Paperwork must be filled out detailing the type of treatment, clinic, costs and other details. Once the paperwork is completed, it goes through the approval process with the concerned dental care insurer. The length of time for approval ranges with each firm.

DENTAL CLAIMS FOR CLIENTS AND CDAnet

CDA(*Canadian Dental Association*) works closely with the Canadian Life & Health Insurance Association (CLHIA) to ensure that dentists' submissions of requests for advance confirmation of coverage comply with privacy legislation.

CDAnet is the most efficient, time-saving and cost-saving method of processing claims, with no sign-up fees (for modem transmission) or transaction costs.

CDAnet Advantages

Processing the dental claims (CDAnet formatted message) electronically:
- Allows carriers to process them and reimburse patients for the covered portion of their treatment more quickly.
- Eliminates delays caused by late or lost mail.
- Reduces the time it takes for patients to be reimbursed for treatment by half.

Carriers can electronically inform dentists that:
- The patient is eligible for coverage
- The recommended procedures are covered
- A pre-determination is required
- There is an error in the claim
- The carrier will pay the amount indicated

CDAnet certified office software reduces or eliminates:
- Paper handling and filing
- Rejected claims (by instantly checking patient and procedure data)
- Waiting time for pre-determinations.

Dental Claims and Payment Policy

The Dental Claims and Payment Policy is offered to dental practices using CDAnet. The dentists are invited to copy or otherwise reproduce below given text for use in their practice. They are advised to place this message on the front desk or in the reception area to ensure that their patients read this Dental Claims and Payment Policy.

Sample Dental Claims and Payment Policy

- *Using CDAnet, this practice is able to transmit your dental claims electronically.*
- *CDAnet transmits your dental claim immediately and speeds up the reimbursement process.*
- *Depending on your plan, you may receive your cheque in less than a week. Our staff will be happy to assist you with the necessary forms, should your dental plan not offer electronic processing.*
- *We will make every effort to help you determine the nature of your dental plan coverage prior to the start of treatment. However, in all cases, the patient is fully responsible for the complete cost of treatment on the day of their appointment. We ask that payment be received at the time of treatment by means of a cheque, cash or credit card.*
- *We also recognize that the cost of treatment can be high for some patients who require major treatment. Our staff is happy to set up payment plans for our regular patients who have established a good payment record with our office.*
- *We thank you for your understanding and continued confidence in the care we give our patients.*

Claims Forms, reimbursement and Co-Payments

Filling out a dental claim form can be a bit of a challenge. There are laws governing how a claim form may be used by an employer or plan provider.

ODA (*Ontario Dental Association*) highlights some important things about privacy protection and security of those covered under dental benefits.

Assignment of Benefits

The "assignment of benefits" is when a dental patient instructs an insurance carrier to make a payment of permissible benefits directly to the dentist.

Active decision-making about oral health care by patients and meaningful involvement in the financial matters of dental care, including the dental plan, is an important part of achieving excellent oral health care.

The **important points and advantages** are as follows:

- The patient may not have to pay the dentist up front, and then go through the process of filing a claim with their insurance carrier and wait to get reimbursed.
- This way an obvious long process can be avoided due to insurance carrier making a payment of permissible benefits directly to the dentist.

- Dental claim reimbursement is much faster than it was years ago, and patients are finding that when they pay the dentist directly their reimbursement cheque is received quickly
- This process greatly minimizing the time they are out of pocket.
- It is not unusual to see the dentist on Monday and have the reimbursement cheque before the end of the week, due to faster way of electronic claims submission.
- Many dentists accept credit cards, which typically have a monthly billing cycle. If complex treatment is necessary, dentists can arrange a payment schedule that allows a patient to budget for expenses and get reimbursement that is more conveniently timed.

Co-Payments
What is co-payment?

Many dental plans have co-payments, or in other words, a percentage of the claim amount that is not covered by the dental plan.Co-payment—also called co-insurance—is the portion of the bill that is client's own responsibility. It is the most common way for dental plans to limit the costs, thereby providing various plans with an assortment of benefits and price points for the purchaser to choose. Some plans are also taking other approaches to limit plan spending: setting annual deductibles, capping the dollar amount or limiting the number of visits covered within a year.

A dental plan covers 80% of the bill where an 80/20 co-payment is common for basic procedures such as x-rays, cleaning, fillings, and root canals. A 50/50 co-payment is common for major procedures such as crowns and bridges. But there are many variations. Depends on their plan, the client has to pay.

Under the Dentistry Act, 1991 (Regulated Health Professions Act) dentists are required to make a reasonable attempt to collect the co-payment portion of dental fees for which the patient has payment responsibility. The profession's regulatory body, the Royal College of Dental Surgeons of Ontario (RCDSO) is responsible for ensuring dentists adhere to this requirement.

Co-payment and professional obligation

The dentist has a professional obligation to collect the co-payment. But it is not easy always. In difficult situations, the term "reasonable" should be noted, by taking into account the circumstances of the situation. This includes occasions when dentist understand that the patient cannot afford to pay the co-payment and the dentist may decide to end pursuing the collection.

The following options are open to make sure that the dental plan administrator is not misled:

1. Citing the reasons why this decision has been made, the dentist can advise the dental plan administrator of the situation and obtain his or her consent in writing to cease attempting to collect the co-payment and;

2. Also stating the reasons why, the dentist could advise the dental plan administrator that he or she does not intend to collect the co-payment, and that he or she will accept as full payment, the amount the plan administrator will pay under the plan.

In such cases, no attempts to mislead the dental plan administrator have been made. Intentional misrepresentation by the dentist can result in discipline by the RCDSO, loss or suspension of dental registration and criminal proceedings for insurance fraud. Evidently, waiving the co-payment and misleading the plan administrator put at risk everyone involved — the dentist, the dental office administrator and the plan sponsor.

Please Pay Subscriber

Printed in capital letters at the top right-hand corner on the ODA Standard Dental Claim Form is a box stamped, "Please Pay Subscriber." It encourages the patient to be an active participant in their dental care, in a system where a plan sponsor and an insurance carrier is involved. By not signing this box, the patient pays the dentist for the care received and then submits the completed claim form to the insurance carrier for reimbursement for the eligible benefit amount. The carrier then pays that amount directly to client, the plan member or subscriber.

If the claim is electronically transmitted by the dental office to the carrier, then the patient may pay the dentist and the carrier will send the reimbursement to the plan member. This process is called non-assignment. Here, the subscriber did not assign his or her insurance benefits to the dentist, nor did the dentist accept assignment. This simple process has far-reaching benefits. The patient is aware of the cost of the dental service and will be more likely to:

- comply with treatment regimens;
- acquire knowledge about the nature and extent of dental benefits;
- become a better consumer of dental care and wise user of dental benefits;
- develop an important comfort level for discussing fees with the dentist;
- identify areas in the design of a dental plan that could be improved and apprise dental plan sponsors in response.

The ODA has a long-standing philosophy encouraging non-assignment dental plans for the simple reason that when patients have a meaningful financial involvement in their dental care, better decisions are made.

Information About Using Claim Forms
Using SIN(Social Insurance Number) as Identification and Privacy Concerns

The patient must provide his or her certification, SIN or identification number in Part 2 of the ODA Standard Dental Claim Form. Patients who are unsure of their identification number should refer to their employee benefits card or consult the Benefits Department at their place of employment.

The standard dental claim form conforms with the Personal Information Protection and electronic Documents Act (PIPEDA), a federal privacy law. The release on the claim form reads as follows:

I understand that the fees listed in this claim may not be covered by or may exceed my plan benefits. I understand that I am financially responsible to my dentist for the entire treatment. I acknowledge that the total fee of $ is accurate and has been charged to me for services rendered.

I authorize the release of information contained in this claim to my ensuring company/plan administrator. I also authorize the communication of information related to the coverage of services described in this form of the named dentist.

The Canadian Dental Association is also amending the standard dental pre-treatment form to reflect the same wording change. Dentists using CDAnet, are also required to update each patient (parent/guardian) signature on file. For each patient participating in CDAnet the following wording must accompany the signature:

I authorize release, to my dental benefit plan administrator and the CDA, information contained in claims submitted electronically. I also authorize the communication of information related to the coverage of services described to the named dentist. This authorization shall continue in effect until the undersigned revokes the same.

Important to know-
- The signature on file must be updated every three years.
- The signature serves two purposes: it authorizes the dentist to submit the claim/estimate electronically and it authorizes the plan administrator to send the electronic explanation of benefits (EOB) or pre-determination of benefits (POB) or claim acknowledgement back to the dental office.
- Dentists are obligated to give the EOB, POB or claim acknowledgment to the patient prior to leaving the office.

Assignment from insurance companies

Some dentists do not accept direct payment (assignment) from insurance companies for certain reasons. Assignment causes problems because the administrative costs of filing claims and collecting partial or full reimbursement from dozens of insurance companies for hundreds of patients places a heavy financial and extremely undesirable administrative burden on a dental practice. In addition to this, many companies and plans are now sending reimbursement to the patients anyway, regardless of whether the claim was assigned to the dentist or not.

According to the *Ontario Dental Association*, these are a some reasons why dentists should stop taking assignment:

· Dentists urged to have dental services exempt from the GST. But, due to GST burden on dental supplies with no reduction in tax credit adds to already rising practice costs. Assignment is expensive and confers very little real benefit to the patient except convenience.

· Credit cards and post-dated cheques allow up to 30 days for payment while insurance company cheques are processed within 3 to 15 days (quicker with e-billing that many offices now offer).

· Clients accepting own claims means they are actively involved in their dental health and are a better informed consumer.

· A great number of dental patients in Ontario already collect payment directly from their insurance companies and report that prompt reimbursement is not a problem.

· Assignment is expensive and a major contributor to practice costs, and rising dental fees and insurance premiums. Eliminating assignment may allow for savings in premiums and dental fees.

DENTAL FINANCING

Dental financing is a payment alternate when a client can not afford to pay for necessary dental care all at once. Dental financing could mean borrowing money to pay for the treatment (may be an expensive one) and then making monthly payments until it is paid off. Financing also typically involves paying fees and interest on the money borrowed.

Dental work is certainly expensive, and many Canadians are unable to cover the cost of some of these procedures. If a client needs dental work done but can't afford to pay for it all on their own, dental financing and dental loans help them decide which dental financing product is right for them and which lender can provide it.

There are situations when a patient/client can not afford a treatment such as-

- Mostly attributed to the high cost of the treatment
- The client does not have dental insurance
- Their dental plan will not cover the treatment

The client can speak with the dental office administrator about dental financing, who may be ready and prepared to assist the client in this matter.

Benefits of Dental financing:

- Dental financing is a flexible payment option that allows patients to get necessary treatments in an affordable manner.

- A customised payment plan can be developed for a client by a dental office administrator so that he/she can only pay what they can afford while still getting the treatment they need.

- The dental financing can help client to avoid the stress and pain from more expensive dental health problems that may worsen over time.

- Direct insurance billing and flexible dental financing options can help clients avoid the pressure of paying for entire dental bills upfront so that they can keep more money in their pockets.

- To get dental insurance and figure out the best plans for the clients and their families, dental office administrator can provide recommendations and a list of the insurance companies they work with for direct billing.

Dental Financing and Dental Loans

Dental financing is typically not collateralized, which means there is nothing of value that is used to back the loan in case you are no longer able to make payments. lenders who provide such loans depend on factors such as your credit score, income, assets, and most recent financial activity to determine what type of borrower you would be.

Dental Work loans are specific types of financing products devised to cover the cost of dental work, including surgery and other procedures. Dental problems are sometimes unique and unpredictable. Dental problems can be their own conditions or may be reflecting an underlying condition. Dental work is sometimes unavoidable may be due to reasons related to pain, esthetic, or preservation of teeth. Whether it is a simple scaling of teeth, a root canal procedure, an elective surgery or a cosmetic teeth build-up, the price is always high. As a matter of fact, dental work can be downright expensive and can often be way out of a client's affordability. When applying for dental work loans, the client can request a specific loan amount required to pay for any dental work they need.

Dental Financing Options

For the clients needing some financial assistance to pay for dental work needed, some of the options are as follows:

Personal loan

Many prefer to use personal loan to pay for their dental work. These loans are generally unsecured, which means no collateral is needed for this type of loan. The interest rate and the loan amount one may be eligible for depends on the strength of their credit and financial health. Personal loans are paid back in installments until the full loan amount – plus interest – is repaid.

A personal loan can be used to pay for a range of personal expenses, which can include dental work and medical treatment. These loans are typically unsecured loans, which mean the lender doesn't require any collateral to secure the loan. Because of this, the lender will typically consider many factors — including your credit history — to determine whether you'll be able to repay the loan. If you've got lower credit scores, you may end up paying higher interest rates or may be denied a loan outright.

Secured personal loan

A secured personal loan is a loan that is backed by an asset. Lenders typically require the client to back the loan with a house. However, some secured loans can also be backed by something other than a house, like a car, for instance.

Credit cards

Credit cards can be used to put the dental treatment costs on it. However, spending a lot on the credit card or if the amount on credit is close to the credit limit may negatively impact individual's credit score. Moreover, credit card there are high-interest rates that come with credit cards.

Medical credit cards

Medical credit cards may be available to pay for healthcare treatments, including dental procedures. They are similar to regular credit card but can only be used to pay for healthcare and only within a certain network of providers that accept the card for medical or dental care. After that, the individual has to make payments to card issuer.

Introductory 0% APR credit card

There are credit cards that offer an introductory 0% APR(annual percentage rate) for purchases and balance transfers for a set period of time. After the introductory period ends, the card will have an APR based on client's credit and other factors. Each intro APR offering can vary based on the lender and individual's credit. However, taking advantage of a 0% offer also has the potential to damage their credit score, too.

Provider financing

Some dentists may also offer the opportunity to apply for payment plans and in-house financing through third-party lenders. Some lenders may offer loans that don't require any money down or that has a low down payment. And others may not require a credit check to be approved. However, they may have high APRs and fees.

In-house financing

Dental work that is more expensive is more likely to come with the option to finance, such as orthodontic braces, cosmetic treatment or dental implants. Many dental offices provide financing programs that allow clients to take out financing directly through their dentist. Many of these programs are interest-free, at least for a specific period of time, after which interest may be charged.

Specialized dental loan

There are specific lenders who offer these types of unique loans. These are certain types of loans that are designed for medical procedures, including dental work. Procedures that are not covered by the provincial health care may be eligible for specialized dental financing. Many of these types of loan programs are also applicable to cosmetic procedures that fall under the scope of dental work.

Line of credit

Line of credit is somewhat similar to a personal loan, but instead of getting a lump sum of money to pay for the dental work, it provides the access to a credit line that one can withdraw funds from as needed. Interest will be charged on the amount taken out.

Dentalcard

Certain companies in Canada and US are offering an array of dental finance programs to the citizens. Dentalcard is one of them. Dentalcard can pre-approve an approximate amount with the flexibility to choose the dentist, service provider, procedure, product purchase or procedure date with the comfort of knowing that financing has been confirmed for a client. A client can submit an application to Dentacard online. Dentalcard will notify the client of the credit decision by phone and sends payment automatically to the selected dentist or service provider.

Dental Procedures can be paid with Dental Financing

The type of dental work that dental financing can cover is vast and can include any of the following:

- Regular Check-ups
- Prophylactic scaling of teeth
- Cosmetic & conservative teeth buildup
- Endodontics-such as RCT
- Periodontics- scaling, gingival & periodontal surgeries
- Fluoride application
- Teeth Restorations
- Preventive measures-Sealants
- Mouthguards
- Dental implants
- Crown & bridge prostheses
- Orthodontic Braces
- Retainers & Invisalign
- Esthetic Lumineers and Veneers
- Bite plates
- Headgear

CHAPTER 31

BANKING AND DENTAL PRACTICE

There are numerous banking services available to small businesses, such as dental offices, and there is considerable competition between financial institutions to acquire and maintain business accounts. Each dental office has at least one commercial or business chequing account. This type of account is known as a current account. Current accounts are intended to be used for commercial purposes which are opened in the name of the business, the dentist, or the dental office.

Patient payment options

Dental clients can choose from a variety of payment options, such as cash, cheque, credit card, debit card or interac-e-transfer. Payments received by mail are entered in the same manner as those made in person. Patients making cash or cheque payments must always be given a receipt. Some patients may wish to leave a postdated cheque to allow time for the insurance payment to be received.

All payments must be entered on the account ledger card and on the daily journal page. Many dental patients choose to pay their account using a credit card, such as MasterCard or VISA. This form of payment provides convenience to patients to allow time for insurance payments to arrive.

DOA and Banking responsibilities

- One of the important daily responsibilities of DOA is to oversee all payments received and to ensure that they are appropriately deposited, while maintaining a consecutive bank balance.
- DOA help to bill and coordinate schedules for patients
- DOA must understand basic bank services
- DOA must know how to write cheques, prepare deposit slips, and reconcile the bank statement monthly
- DOA need to have knowledge to control the bank account
- Maintain the dental clinic's budget, general ledger and accounting systems
- Oversee the processing of insurance and secondary insurance claims
- Assist patients with applying for credit and other financial assistance

Accounts receivable in Dental office

Accounting and bookkeeping services are very important aspects within a dental practice and good knowledge of account receivable and accounts payables is beneficial for a successful dental practice. Additionally, dental team understands that field of dentistry gets constant change accompanied with growing competition.

Account receivables represent money that is owed to the practice for services that have been rendered. Accounts Receivable is an ASSET that loses its value rapidly. It doesn't matter how much you are billing if you don't collect the fees for your services. Accounts Receivable represent services that you have already provided for which you deserve to be compensated in a timely manner. As a dental Office Administrator, you should inform the patient of the financial policy of the office as well as the payment options available to them. You should not lose a client because of their inability to pay. A healthy dental office is believed to have an accounts-receivable ratio of 1.0, meaning the total accounts receivable are equal to the average monthly production. This accounts-receivable ratio is figured by dividing your total accounts receivable by your average monthly production.

Important points

- It is better to have little or no accounts receivable and steady cash flow
- Uncontrolled Accounts receivable dramatically impacts your cash flow in a negative way
- The main success factor to collections is the role of entire dental team who needs to believe in the quality of the services performed and the fairness of the fees charged.
- If anyone in the team does not support the financial policies of the office and follow through with recommended procedures, he/she may turn out to be a liability to the practice.
- You must have sufficient cash flow to pay your bills, such as payroll
- Bad habits develop quickly, and you may not notice
- DOA and also other team members must be capable of discussing fees and payment options with patients.

Collection Letters

Typically, a collection letter is sent when a debtor's invoice has become past-due. Financially, this means that the consumer has fallen behind with his regular payments and owes a certain amount to the lender. The client in a dental office who receives a collection letter knows that their account is overdue and knows why they are receiving the letter.

Collection letters can be a as follows-
- Reminder Collection Letter- written with an assumption that customer forgets to make the payment.
- Inquiry Collection Letter- As the name suggests, the main purpose of this type of

letter is to make an inquiry regarding the payment.
- Appeal collection Letter.
- Ultimatum Collection Letter.

All collection letters should be phrased in firm, positive, business-like terms that make every effort to persuade the patient to pay the debt, to help them pay it and to enable them to save face while doing so.

Collection Agencies and Unpaid accounts

Patients are unfortunately not always responsive to simple phone systems and online payment portals. At that point, it is time to step in and contact them using out collection services. Then, they will be more likely to pay in a swift manner to ensure they are out of debt. Many companies provide customized medical and dental debt recovery processes to help the dental practice. Unpaid accounts can be referred for collection while there is still hope of settlement, usually no more than three months after the end of treatment. The collection agency should be given all information that may be helpful and should be kept informed on any new information. The agency should also be notified promptly if the patient pays directly to the dental office.

Accounts payable in Dental office and DOA

Accounts payable (AP) represents the amount that a company owes to its creditors and suppliers (also referred to as a current liability account). Accounts payable is recorded on the balance sheet under current liabilities.

There are two main types of expenses:
1. Fixed expenses- include costs, such as rent, utilities, and salaries that go on whether or not the dentist is in the office and whether or not professional services are actually being provided.
2. Variable expenses- include those expenses that change depending upon the type of services rendered and the amount consumed such as sundry supplies, laboratory fees, and repairs.

The effective management of a dental office requires organized handling and prompt payment of all bills for practice-related expenses. It is important for the dental office administrator to be knowledgeable about single entry bookkeeping and related tasks such as writing cheques, making bank deposits, and maintaining petty cash records. Most major expense payments are handled by writing a cheque and posting the entry to the appropriate expense category in a disbursements journal.

Some dentists prefer for the DOA to pay the bills as they are incurred; others prefer to wait until the supplier's statement is received. Accuracy is essential, however, so the DOA should try to select a specific time with no or a few distractions. Accurate inventory control is essential to managing the office expenses. The control system should be maintained and updated at all times. As such the budget for clinical consumable supplies should not exceed 5-7% of gross production per month. As productivity increases, the budget can adjust accordingly. An efficient and competent DOA knows that the best way to reduce expenses is to increase revenue, though.

Payroll Considerations and dental practice

In most dental practices the dental office administrator is the person responsible for the appropriate and accurate administration of payroll and staff remuneration duties. It is crucial to maintain accurate and complete records of the hours worked, deductions, and government remittances while completing payroll work. It is also vital to protect the confidential nature of the client records. Time records should be kept for all part-time, hourly, and salaried employees including regular, overtime, and vacation hours, as well as weekend shifts and holidays.

As per the federal and provincial taxation requirements and guidelines, source deductions are subtracted from the gross earnings of every employee. The gross pay is the rate of pay before deductions are withheld. The pay that remains after deductions is called the net pay. DOA should have the basic information about gross pay and net pay of all employees if they are appointed for the payroll duties. All employee deductions including the employer's portion must be remitted to the Receiver General by the 15th of the subsequent month.

All employers must withhold the following deductions:

- Income tax
- Canada Pension Plan contribution (CPP)
- Employment insurance (EI) premiums.

Deductions should be taken according to the rules and regulations stated in the Employer's Guide to Payroll Deductions, available from Revenue Canada. It is important for the DOA to be aware of the rules and regulations regarding the insurability of earnings. The regulations affect the amount of deductions taken from the employee, as well as the employer's contribution. An employer is responsible for submitting 1.4 times the amount of the employee's premiums on insurable earnings for the pay period. A Canada Pension Plan deduction is taken from all earnings, provided that the employee is over 18 years of age and under 70 years of age, up to an annual maximum specified in the Payroll Deduction Tables from Revenue Canada.

Generally new Tax Deductions Tables are sent to each employer by January 1 each year. They are also accessible on the Internet by going to http://www.cra-arc.gc.ca.

PD7A Forms and T4 Slips

As per the trend of electronic transactions, CRA has launched a new program to allow practice to receive your PD7A form online. The PD7A, usually a two- or three-part form, is mailed to the dental office automatically each month. The Employer Number or account number appears on each section of the form. This number identifies the employer to Revenue Canada. There are spaces available to record the details of the remittance such as tax deductions, CPP contributions, and EI premiums, along with the total amount of the remittance. The month in which the deductions were made will be displayed in the third section under "Month for which deductions were withheld."

Every employer is required to online submit or forward completed T4 Supplementary and related T4 Summary forms to the appropriate taxation centre, on or before the last day of February each year for the preceding calendar year.

Please note the terms **CLIENT** and **PATIENT** are used interchangeably throughout the book. **It means the same.**

(**EXPLANATION-***The definition of a client is a person or group that uses the professional advice or services of a lawyer, accountant, advertising agency, architect, etc. A patient is a person who is under medical care or treatment. As per views of many, most modern dentistry requires an out-of-pocket expense, requiring discretionary decisions about time and money. Hence, the people being diagnosed and treated are clients. However, they should be considered patients as dental procedures/operations are performed on them.*)

ABOUT THE AUTHOR

Prof. Usha Dabas

Prof (Dr.) Usha Dabas is a Healthcare Professional, Educationist and Author with over 30 years of academic, clinical and administrative expertise in the fields of Medicine, Dentistry and Healthcare. She has authored nearly 10 Textbooks on the general and specialty subject matters of Medical and Dental Health Science. She is Director, Healthcare Faculty at Springfield College of Healthcare, Ontario, Canada. She had also worked in various Medical and Dental Universities across the globe in high academic positions and has earned laurel through her educational expertise.

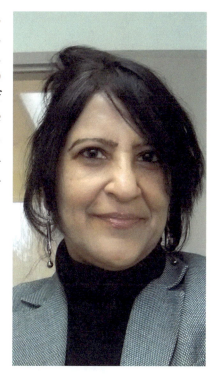

OTHER BOOKS BY THE SAME AUTHOR

Dental Billing, Coding & Insurance in Canadian Dental Office Administration: with current updates

This book is a compilation of important topics related to dental billing & coding, dental insurance, dental claims and related procedures in Canadian dental office administration with most current developments and updated information. The book discusses in detail the crucial components of a successful dental office practice with primary focus upon newly introduced Canada Government Aided Dental Coverage-CDCP program, its application in daily practice, Non-Insured Health Benefits Programs (NIHB), Interim Federal Health Program (IFHP), Schedule of Benefits (SOB), dental plans and dental financing, dental claims for clients and CDAnet, role of dental team and efficient engagement of stakeholders in dentistry.

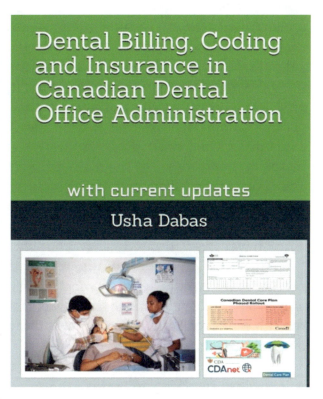

Ethics And Law in Dental & Medical Sciences

This book is intended to provide dental office professionals and administrators an important insight into the ethics, law and ethico-legal aspects of the modern-day dentistry, and also understanding of how to deal with these issues that they encounter in their daily dental practice. In the modern times, with technological advancements taking place by leaps and bounds, dental office professionals and administrators must familiarize themselves with the prevailing laws, regulations, and standards that affect their professional decisions in their clinical practice. The knowledge and information conveyed in the book is expected to help understand ethical, legal and professional responsibility and promote ethical conduct in the field of dentistry. It also focuses upon common ethical dilemmas and legal issues and their solutions. The book is intended to provide aspiring students and dental office professionals ethicolegal teaching guide with a set of values that they can carry into their workplaces and modern society having diversity in cultural and ethnical beliefs, with the definite standards of principles and ideals.

Dental Fundamentals for Auxiliary Staff: A Book for Dental Office Administrators

This book is regarded by the author as an introduction to modern dentistry and its fundamental concepts obligatory to an accurate dental practice. The text is written primarily to aid dental staff members, who are not merely engaged but truly serve as the essential segment of the modern-day dental practice such as dental administrators, dental hygienists, dental technicians, dental nurses and dental surgery assistants. This book deals from the fundamental and historical background of the dentistry to the current trends and future of the dentistry. All the concepts are compiled to highlight the most recent advancements in the sphere of Oral and dental science. This book will be very useful for all those who have ever desired and cherished to learn the fundamentals and perceptions of dentistry as well as participate as an effective team member in the dental office. It will also provide guidance to the new entrants to understand the subject of Oral and dental science thoroughly, faster and more effectively.

Advances in Dentistry: A Series

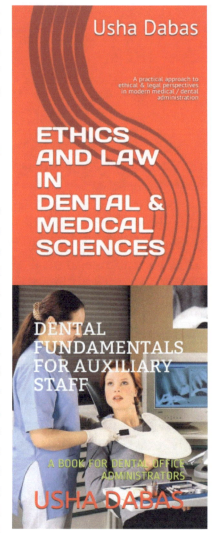

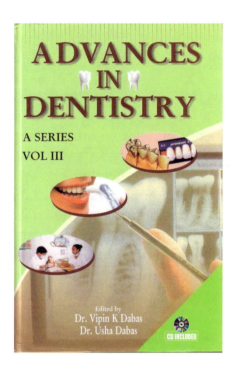

Anxiety & Depression - A Journey from Suffering to Thriving

This is a motivational and inspiring story of a mental health warrior, a medical professional herself, and sufferer of the severe anxiety, depression, and stress, who kept fighting, beat her all odds and finally emerged victorious through her determination and resolve. The story in the book has been written in the narrator's own words to keep its purity and appeal. This can be the story of everyone living on this planet, however, as we keep facing our demons every day in diverse life conditions. Life is full of experiences of happy and sad moments. Trauma, agonies, positivity, negativity, pain, success, and failure are integral parts of life. At times, they confound our minds to the extent that minds get overwhelmed and baffled in dealing with them. This may culminate into different forms of psychological expression or mental illness such as anxiety, depression, PTSD, or panic attacks. Our mental health can destroy us. "YOUR MIND IS THE WORST ENEMY OF YOURS"—the sufferers of mental

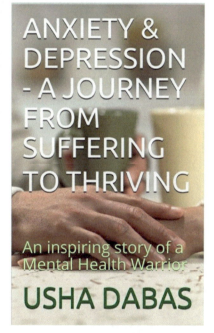

health agree to the fact due to their physical and mental struggle for survival and dealing with stigma. Through this book, the author emphasizes that it is crucial to talk about mental health. Talking about mental health provides us opportunity to seek help, find people who can relate and connect, and step toward wellbeing.

The Deaths, lived all the way through: Based upon True Incidents

'The Deaths, lived all the way through'- is a collection of stories revolving around physical loss and emotional trauma associated with the loss of someone close or an integral part of one's life. The book through all the stories conveys the message that there is some important connection between death and 'the meaning of life'. The book focuses on the concept of universal connection that nothing in the world stands by itself. Every object is a link in an endless chain and is thus connected with all other links. The book also philosophically explains that the fear of death is only natural to humans, but death should be viewed as the achievement of life too.

Very moving, emotive and touching stories -Must read for everyone.

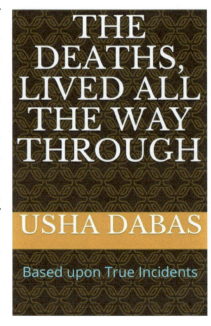

Surviving Honor killing- A Chronicle of women Hatred, oppression and abuse (Hindi Edition)

This book is a very well-written, captivating narrative of a woman hatred, cruelty and abuse. This honor killing survivor's story is a shocking tale of woman-to-woman rivalry, focusing upon disgraceful struggle of power and cultural belief to consider the women as objects and commodities, and not as human beings endowed with dignity and rights.

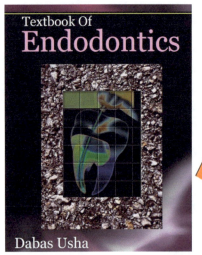
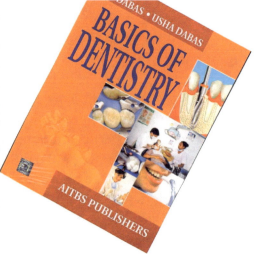
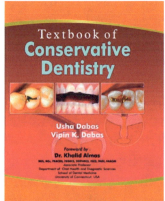

Manufactured by Amazon.ca
Bolton, ON

45165035R00116